Contemporary Surgical Clerkships

Series Editor
Adam E. M. Eltorai, Marlborough, USA

This series of specialty-specific books will serve as high-yield, quick-reference reviews specifically for the numerous third- and fourth-year medical students rotating on surgical clerkships. Edited by experts in the field, each book includes concise review content from a senior resident or fellow and an established academic physician. Students can read the text from cover to cover to gain a general foundation of knowledge that can be built upon when they begin their rotation, or they can use specific chapters to review a subspecialty before starting a new rotation or seeing a patient with a subspecialty attending.

These books will be the ideal, on-the-spot references for medical students and practitioners seeking fast facts on diagnosis and management. Their bullet-pointed format, including user-friendly figures, tables and algorithms, make them the perfect quick-reference. Their content breadth covers the most commonly encountered problems in practice, focusing on the fundamental principles of diagnosis and management. Carry them in your white coat for convenient access to the answers you need, when you need them.

James A. Madura II • David G. Pearson
Natasha A. Sioda
Editors

Bariatric Surgery Clerkship

A Guide for Senior Medical Students

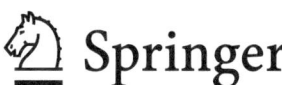

Editors
James A. Madura II
Chair, Division of General Surgery
Mayo Clinic Hospital
Phoenix, AZ, USA

David G. Pearson
Department of Surgery
Mayo Clinic Hospital
Phoenix, AZ, USA

Natasha A. Sioda
General Surgery Resident
Mayo Clinic Hospital
Phoenix, AZ, USA

Editorial Contact: Jessica Chio

ISSN 2730-941X ISSN 2730-9428 (electronic)
Contemporary Surgical Clerkships
ISBN 978-3-031-92963-2 ISBN 978-3-031-92964-9 (eBook)
https://doi.org/10.1007/978-3-031-92964-9

© Mayo Foundation for Medical Education and Research, a Minnesota charitable corporation 2025

This work is subject to copyright. All rights are solely and exclusively licensed by the Publisher, whether the whole or part of the material is concerned, specifically the rights of translation, reprinting, reuse of illustrations, recitation, broadcasting, reproduction on microfilms or in any other physical way, and transmission or information storage and retrieval, electronic adaptation, computer software, or by similar or dissimilar methodology now known or hereafter developed.

The use of general descriptive names, registered names, trademarks, service marks, etc. in this publication does not imply, even in the absence of a specific statement, that such names are exempt from the relevant protective laws and regulations and therefore free for general use.

The publisher, the authors and the editors are safe to assume that the advice and information in this book are believed to be true and accurate at the date of publication. Neither the publisher nor the authors or the editors give a warranty, expressed or implied, with respect to the material contained herein or for any errors or omissions that may have been made. The publisher remains neutral with regard to jurisdictional claims in published maps and institutional affiliations.

This Springer imprint is published by the registered company Springer Nature Switzerland AG
The registered company address is: Gewerbestrasse 11, 6330 Cham, Switzerland

If disposing of this product, please recycle the paper.

Contents

1 **Epidemiology of Obesity**................................. 1
  Grace Madura, Benjamin Veenstra, and Natasha A. Sioda

2 **History of Bariatric Surgery** 5
  Marlene Garcia-Neuer, Benjamin Veenstra, and Natasha A. Sioda

3 **Physiology of Obesity and Obesity Related Diseases**............... 15
  Sneha Mishra and Natasha A. Sioda

4 **Pre-operative Preparation for Bariatric Surgery** 21
  Natasha A. Sioda, Benjamin Veenstra, John Timothy Prior,
  John Raynak, and Narjeet Khurmi

5 **Bariatric Technique and Outcomes**........................... 35
  Nisha Rehman, David G. Pearson, Sinong Qian, Nicholas Nolan,
  Holly Grossman, and Natasha A. Sioda

6 **Post-operative Complications Following Bariatric Surgery** 55
  Lena Egbert, James A. Madura II, Aaron Munoz, Natasha A. Sioda,
  and Fernando Elli

7 **Alternatives to Bariatric Surgery** 77
  Isabella Reitz, Fernando Elli, Lindsey Trinchet,
  and Natasha A. Sioda

Index.. 91

Chapter 1
Epidemiology of Obesity

Grace Madura, Benjamin Veenstra, and Natasha A. Sioda

Introduction

Obesity is a diagnosis based on the Body Mass Index (BMI) a value calculated by taking the patient's weight in kilograms divided by the square of the patient's height in meters. The World Health Organization classifies a BMI of 25–29.9 to be considered overweight and a BMI over 30 to be obese [1].

Incidence and Prevalence

- Over 2 billion adults worldwide were estimated to have obesity in 2022 [2].
- Increasing rates of childhood obesity, with an estimated 160 million children and adolescents aged 5–19 with obesity worldwide
- Prevalence is higher in women than men in all age brackets [3].
- Obesity is most prevalent in ages 60–64 in women and 50–54 in men

---

G. Madura
Mayo Clinic Alix School of Medicine, Scottsdale, AZ, USA
e-mail: madura.grace@mayo.edu

B. Veenstra
Mayo Clinic, Jacksonville, FL, USA
e-mail: veenstra.benjamin@mayo.edu

N. A. Sioda (✉)
Mayo Clinic, Phoenix, AZ, USA
e-mail: sioda.natasha@mayo.edu

© The Author(s), under exclusive license to Springer Nature Switzerland AG 2025
J. A. Madura II et al. (eds.), *Bariatric Surgery Clerkship*, Contemporary Surgical Clerkships, https://doi.org/10.1007/978-3-031-92964-9_1

- In the US, the prevalence of obesity was estimated to be 41.9% as part of the National Health and Nutrition Examination Survey in 2017–2020 [4].
- Non-Hispanic black adults had a higher prevalence of obesity compared to Hispanic and non-Hispanic white populations in the US [4].

Growing Epidemic

Obesity rates have increased since the early 1980s [5].

- Prevalence has doubled in many countries of various sociodemographic indices

Contributing factors to increasing rates of obesity have been suggested such as:

- Energy-dense, processed foods [6]
- Increased supply and access to food
- Increased food marketing
- Decreased physical activity in built and urban environments

Obesity is associated with many disease states including:

- Cardiovascular disease [3]
- Type 2 Diabetes Mellitus
- Chronic kidney disease
- Cancer
- Musculoskeletal disorders

The increased prevalence and healthcare burden of obesity has inspired many international task forces to further characterize health impacts, create health policy, and guide treatment. Despite numerous guidelines, the treatment of obesity continues to challenge healthcare providers today.

References

1. Obesity: preventing and managing the global epidemic. Report of a WHO consultation. World Health Organ Tech Rep Ser. 2000;894:i–253.
2. World Health Organization (WHO). Obesity and overweight. https://www.who.int/news-room/fact-sheets/detail/obesity-and-overweight. Published 1 March 2024.
3. GBD 2015 Obesity Collaborators, Afshin A, Forouzanfar MH, et al. Health effects of overweight and obesity in 195 countries over 25 years. N Engl J Med. 2017;377(1):13–27. https://doi.org/10.1056/NEJMoa1614362.

4. Stierman B, Afful J, Carroll MD, et al. National Health and Nutrition Examination Survey 2017–March 2020 prepandemic data files—development of files and prevalence estimates for selected health outcomes. 2021 June 14. In: National Health Statistics reports [internet]. Hyattsville (MD): National Center for Health Statistics (US); 2024. p. 158.
5. Swinburn BA, Kraak VI, Allender S, et al. The global syndemic of obesity, undernutrition, and climate change: the lancet commission report [published correction appears in Lancet. 2019 Feb 23;393(10173):746. doi:10.1016/S0140-6736(19)30384-8]. Lancet. 2019;393(10173):791–846. https://doi.org/10.1016/S0140-6736(18)32822-8.
6. Swinburn BA, Sacks G, Hall KD, McPherson K, Finegood DT, Moodie ML, Gortmaker SL. The global obesity pandemic: shaped by global drivers and local environments. Lancet. 2011;378(9793):804–14. https://doi.org/10.1016/S0140-6736(11)60813-1. PMID: 21872749.

Chapter 2
History of Bariatric Surgery

Marlene Garcia-Neuer, Benjamin Veenstra, and Natasha A. Sioda

Introduction

The history of bariatric surgery is critical to the practicing general and bariatric surgeon today. Not only does an overview demonstrate the 'why' and 'how' of previous procedures, it also demonstrates the scientific component of surgery and how surgery has contributed to our understanding of nutrition, malabsorption and restriction. Although many of these procedures are no longer practiced today, it is important for surgeons to understand the anatomy since there are still patients who have undergone these procedures and may have complications or require revisions.

We can divide bariatric surgery then into three subsets: malabsorptive, restrictive and metabolic/hormonal [1].

These three options rose and fell in popularity based on our scientific understanding of nutrition and obesity as well as the adverse effects seen after each new procedure.

M. Garcia-Neuer · N. A. Sioda (✉)
Mayo Clinic, Phoenix, AZ, USA
e-mail: garcia-neuer.marlene@mayo.edu; sioda.natasha@mayo.edu

B. Veenstra
Mayo Clinic, Jacksonville, FL, USA
e-mail: veenstra.benjamin@mayo.edu

Malabsorptive Procedures

In the early 1940s and 1950s little was known about the absorptive mechanisms of the small intestine. However, surgeons were becoming experienced with weight loss as a consequence of massive small-bowel resections for trauma, volvulus, hernia or mesenteric ischemia.

Jejunal Ileal Bypass

- In the early 1950s, multiple surgeons started experimenting with malabsorptive procedures for weight loss.
- Dr. Victor Hendrickson of Sweden published the first malabsorptive bariatric procedure by resecting 105 cm of small bowel for weight loss in 1952. Unfortunately, the patient did not lose any weight after the procedure [2].
- In an effort to advance Hendrick's results: both Dr. Richard Varco and Dr. Albert Kremmen in 1953 and 1954, respectively performed jejunal ileal bypasses (JIB) at the University of Minnesota [3].
- The JIB had a critical component that Hendrick's resection did not have: *reversibility* which was essential in order to provide a safe retreat from a potential iatrogenic catastrophe.
- Dr. Kremmen had been studying bowel resection in dogs and reported that resection of a controlled length of small intestine resulted in impaired fat absorption and consequent weight loss.
- Based on these experiments he offered a jejunal ileal bypass to a patient who was unable to maintain her weight loss despite having completed multiple weight loss programs.
- He anastomosed 40 cm proximal jejunum to the distal 10 cm ileum creating a limited channel of intestine that was exposed to the nutrient stream.
- The patient did have a sustained 35 lb. weight loss, however she developed multiple complications which would later be a hallmark of this procedure. Two years after surgery she had an upper gastrointestinal hemorrhage which required vagotomy and pyloroplasty and repeated episodes of bleeding finally requiring Billroth I hemigastrectomy 11 years later. Even after these complications and further surgeries the patient's weight loss was felt to be inadequate and therefore she had a revision to extend the bypass which resulted in a sustained 100 lb. weight loss [3, 4].
- Overall, the JIB procedure was effective for weight loss (patients lost a mean of 58 kg at the end of the first year) [5] however the JIB was also associated with severe complications.
- Anaerobic bacterial overgrowth in the long excluded blind loop, termed "bypass enteritis", caused abdominal distention and lactose intolerance and contributed

to the foul-smelling flatus and stool. Absorption of the bacterial toxins resulted in polyarthralgia and hepatic failure. Continuous diarrhea resulted in anal excoriation and hemorrhoids. Alterations to luminal absorption of fatty acids and calcium lead to increased incidence of nephrolithiasis and renal failure. Loss of potassium, calcium and magnesium, as well as vitamin and protein deficiency resulted in secondary neuropathy, bone demineralization, myalgias and peripheral weakness and edema.

- Over time bowel adaptive changes increased the capacity to absorb carbohydrates despite the continued protein malnutrition and malabsorption of vitamins and minerals [3, 6–8]. Only one third of patients had a benign course. Additionally, here was a 4% mortality in the first two post-operative years, mostly related to acute liver failure [3, 5]. In light of these devastating consequences jejunal ileal bypass was abandoned.

Restrictive Procedures

Significant metabolic complications observed with both intestinal and gastric bypass directed surgeons' attention towards restriction. Surgeons observed that extensive gastric resection with a Billroth 2 anastomosis for peptic ulcer disease and vagotomy produced significant weight loss. This led surgeons to look towards altering gastric anatomy to restrict caloric intake and induce early satiety [8, 9]. Some of the perceived benefits of restrictive operations were the comparative rapidity of performing the procedure over more time intensive bypasses, arguments that they were more physiologic, and minimized malnutrition and its devastating complications.

- The first purely restrictive surgery was performed by Mason and Printen in 1971. The procedure consisted of horizontal division of the upper stomach, creating a small upper pouch that was connected to that gastric fundus via a small conduit, about 1.0–1.5 cm wide along the greater curvature of the stomach, thus maintaining stomach continuity and normal anatomy [10].
- Unfortunately the success was transient and the unsatisfactory weight loss and/or regain was believed to be secondary to staple line dehiscence and/or dilation of pouch and conduit [4]. Pouch dilation and breakdown of the channel continued to plague restrictive gastroplasty.
- Mason continued in his search, believing that sustained gastric restriction could be an effective, low risk and reversible bariatric procedure [4]. This resulted in the vertical band gastroplasty (VBG) [11].
- The procedure consisted of creating a vertical pouch oriented along the proximal lesser curve and separated from the fundus by a staple partition. The size of the pouch and stoma were standardized to 50 mL and 1–2 cm respectively. The outlet of the pouch was then reinforced with a narrow band of polypropylene mesh that was passed through a window created by circular stapler [12]. Although

initially popular and effective with an average weight loss of 30 kg in the first 1 year, only about 20% of patients had sustained weight loss, with approximately 20% requiring bariatric re-operation for inadequate weight loss, esophagitis, band erosion or frequent vomiting [11–15]. In light of the high rate of revision and conversion to other procedures the VBG declined in popularity [4, 12].

Gastric Band

Gastric banding built on the legacy of Mason's vertical band gastroplasty and Laws' Silastic band as a minimally invasive way of creating and maintaining gastric restriction.

- In the early 1970s, Wilkinson experimented with gastric banding, he started with 3–0 Prolene sutures around the greater curvature of the stomach that were snugly inverted with a 1 cm bougie transversing the stomach. He did have weight loss, however this only lasted 3–4 months before the stomach returned to its original size. He then tried a similar approach using propylene mesh to invert the stomach. He trialed this for the first time in 1976. The patient initially had a 60 lb. weight loss. However, after a year the weight loss was not maintained, and they required a conversion to gastric bypass [16].
- He later published a case series of 100 patients that underwent a Nissen fundoplication along with his gastric wrapping to decrease postoperative reflux. He found that he had satisfactory weight loss and gave patients early satiety without any metabolic or physiologic changes. However, weight regain was an issue. Patients developed maladaptive behaviors turning to high calorie liquid foods [16, 17].
- As the operation gained popularity and success, different sizes and materials of mesh were used to decrease inflammation and the potential for erosion. Additionally, the wraps became smaller at 1–2.5 cm across the proximal stomach creating a small upper pouch with a narrow channel to the remaining stomach [9, 18].
- However, these non-adjustable banding procedures ultimately were phased out due to the difficult time creating the correct stoma size and slippage of the stomach either anteriorly or posteriorly through the band. Other complications included band erosions and strictures which led to intractable vomiting, severe food intolerances and esophageal dilation. Finally, like with all other purely restrictive procedures, the pouches would gradually dilate and lead to weight gain and the frequency of reoperations were high for obstruction, reflux esophagitis and intractable vomiting [9, 18].
- At this time Australian surgeon Szinicz was experimenting with an *adjustable* gastric band in rabbits. He lined the silicone rings with a balloon on its undersurface which was attached to a subcutaneous port that could be accessed and adjust the stoma size by adding or removing saline [19].

- Surgeons to develop and bring this concept into clinical practice with Hallberg and Forsell describing their experience in Sweden in 1985 and Kuzmak publishing his results in the United states 1986 [20].
- These adjustable silastic bands provided patients with a variable size stoma that can be altered to maximize weight loss and minimize side effects of restriction like severe food intolerance or esophagitis. Kuzmak demonstrated superior weight loss and fewer complications for the adjustable bands compared to their fixed band counterparts [20].
- The adjustable bands easily displaced the nonadjustable in popularity. Around this time in the early 1990s, laparoscopy was gaining traction and in 1993, Belachew and coworkers described laparoscopic adjustable silicone band placement [21]. The laparoscopic gastric band became the most common bariatric operation in Europe and later the United States. This procedure provided a less invasive and reversible operation with similar *short-term* weight loss compared to gastric bypass or similar procedures.
- However, the pitfalls of this minimally invasive and reversible option included a relatively high rate of complications including band prolapse, esophageal dilation, erosions of the gastric lumen, strictures. And like other restrictive procedures weight loss was not sustained. Although still available, this operation has fallen out of favor [21–23].

Gastric Sleeve

The sleeve gastrectomy was originally described by Marceau in 1993 as part of a biliopancreatic diversion but was not used as a standalone restrictive procedure but rather as a supplement to the duodenal ileal anastomosis. The standalone gastric sleeve became a mainstay through two independent pathways, both as a simplification of the magenstrasse and mill procedure and as a staging procedure for Roux-en-Y gastric bypass [24–28].

- The magenstrasse and mill procedure was invented by Johnston as his simplification to the vertical band gastroplasty (VBG). Johnston's goal was to create a restricted gastric reservoir without implantation of foreign material. Johnston's gastroplasty created a narrow tube along the lesser curvature of the stomach (longer than that of the VBG) along with a circularly stapled hole in the stomach located more distally, just beyond the incisura angularis. The outlet into the antrum was not wrapped in mesh to avoid erosion or stenosis, as seen in the VBG [24].
- The stoma was then created by stapling just lateral and parallel to the lesser curve from the doughnut hole up to the angle of His around a prepositioned bougie. The magenstrasse, or "street of the stomach", conveyed the restricted volume of food from the esophagus to the antral "mill", where normal antral grinding of solid food would take place. Normal gastric emptying was then regulated by an

intact and functioning pylorus. At first, a 40-French bougie was used, but, because of unsatisfactory weight loss, the size was reduced incrementally, and they found that a 32-French bougie resulted in a 63% excess weight loss at 3 years [24].
- Over years, this procedure was simplified to increase weight loss maintenance and decrease risks of the procedure. The circular hole was omitted and instead the staple line began on the greater curve 5–6 cm of the pylorus and sequentially along the bougie [25].
- This simplified the procedure and decreased the risk of gastric fistula formation from the staple line on the greater curve of the stomach as well as decreasing the weight regain from food reflux up into the lateral stomach reservoir. However, this modification did require resection of part of the stomach along with division of the short gastrics which made it a *permanent* procedure. Unfortunately, this new technique came with an increased leak rate specifically around the staple line at the gastroesophageal junction. Part of this was believed to be because the size of the bougie that was used was smaller than the esophagus and therefore the staple line was encroaching on the esophagus. To overcome this, surgeons began veering the last staple load application to the left leaving a small triangular pouch of stomach near the esophagus which helped decrease the risk of leaks [9, 27].
- At the same time Ragean and Granger were performing a two-stage biliary pancreatic diversion (BPD) or Roux-en-Y gastric bypass (RYGB) in the super obese. The aim was to perform the SG, which was technically less challenging than BPD or RYG, and after adequate weight loss returning for definitive procedure. Many of these patients lost enough weight with the sleeve that the secondary procedure was often not pursued or thought to be unnecessary, and thus became a stand-alone procedure for many patients [28–30].

Combination Malabsorptive and Restrictive Procedures

Biliopancreatic Diversion

Because of the morbidity associated with the defunctionalized limb in the jejunoileal procedures, Scopinaro and colleagues of Genoa, Italy developed the biliopancreatic diversion (BPD) procedure in the mid-1970s.

- The procedure involved a partial distal gastrectomy with closure of the duodenal stump. The jejunum was divided 250 cm proximal to the ileocecal valve. The distal limb (Roux limb) was then anastomosed to the proximal stomach. The proximal limb (biliopancreatic limb) was anastomosed to the ileum 50 cm proximal to the ileocecal valve. The result was a Roux-en-Y version of the JIB [26, 29, 30].

- Although the biliopancreatic limb was not part of the alimentary channel, conveyance of bile and gastropancreatic juices prevented bacterial overgrowth and thus eliminated the blind loop syndrome of the JIB. The resulting 200-cm Roux limb and 50-cm common channel allowed for rapid transit of food and minimal contact time with digestive enzymes, thereby greatly reducing caloric and nutrient absorption. The partial gastrectomy introduced a restrictive component to the procedure that was believed to enhance the overall initial weight loss achieved. The long-term maintenance of weight loss was attributed to the jejunoileal bypass portion of the procedure.
- The incidence of most of these side effects were greatly reduced with close lifelong follow-up, early detection, intervention, and even prevention [31–34].

Roux-en-Y Gastric Bypass

Mason developed a gastric bypass in 1967, he observed that weight loss was common in patients who underwent gastrectomy for ulcer disease, then studied gastroenterostomy and dogs and concluded that suboptimal gastric bypass could be used for obesity treatment in humans [30–35]. This was essentially a modification to the Billroth II resection but with a different goal. Overall studies showed satisfactory and sustained weight-loss, but the Mason loop was technically difficult and was plagued by bile reflux [36].

- In 1977 Griffith faced this problem by replacing the loop gastrojejunostomy with Roux-en-Y gastric bypass. Roux-en-Y configuration lessened tension on the anastomosis, decreased bile reflux into the pouch and added a malabsorptive component to the operation [37–39].
- To date this is one of the most popular bariatric procedures, with meaningful and sustained weight loss, and dramatic benefits associated with metabolic conditions such as type 2 diabetes. It does still have some of the associated symptoms including dumping syndrome strictures, obstruction, internal hernias, ulcer formation, anastomotic leak, vitamin deficiencies, anemia and in some cases poor weight loss [9, 38].
- Probably one of the greatest advances in all metabolic surgery has been the ability to perform these procedures laparoscopically. Tremblay performed the first laparoscopic Roux-en-Y gastric bypass in 1994 and revolutionized the field [39]. Laparoscopic metabolic surgery improved many perioperative issues including enhancing patient recovery, reducing wound related complications, postoperative pain, hospital stay length, frequency of incisional hernias and mortality [39, 40].

Conclusion

The history and evolution of bariatric surgery is intimately tied history of general abdominal surgery, as well as our understanding of nutrition and metabolism. Surgical management of obesity has evolved over the past 5 decades and now is a popular treatment method for morbidly obese patients. Although many of these procedures or are no longer performed due to severe complications, there are still many patients alive today who are under surveillance for these procedures or are being evaluated for revision. As such, it is important for training and in practice to have a solid understand of the anatomy and the rationale behind these procedures.

References

1. Buchuald H. Metabolic surgery: a brief history and perspective. Surg Obes Relat Dis. 2010;6:221–2.
2. Moshiri M, Osman S, Robinson TJ, Khandelwal S, Bhargava P, Rohrmann CA. Evolution of bariatric surgery: a historical perspective. Am J Roentgenol. 2013;201(1):W40–8.
3. Baker MT. The history and evolution of bariatric surgical procedures. Surg Clin North Am. 2011;91(6):1181–201.
4. Linner J. Early history of bariatric surgery. Surg Obes Relat Dis. 2007;3:569–70.
5. Singh D, Laya AS, Clarkston WK, Allen MJ. Jejunoileal bypass: a surgery of the past and a review of its complications. World J Gastroenterol. 2009;15(18):2277–9.
6. Deitel M. Overview of operations for morbid obesity. World J Surg. 1998;22:913–8.
7. Herbert C. Intestinal bypass for obesity. Can Fam Physician. 1975;21:56–9.
8. Fobi MA. Surgical treatment of obesity: a review. J Natl Med Assoc. 2004;96:61–75.
9. Celio AC, Pories WJ. A history of bariatric surgery: the maturation of a medical discipline. Surg Clin North Am. 2016;96(4):655–67.
10. Printen KJ, Mason EE. Gastric surgery for relief of morbid obesity. Arch Surg. 1973;106(4):428–31.
11. Mason EE. Vertical banded gastroplasty for obesity. Arch Surg. 1982;117(5):701–6.
12. Marsk R, Jonas E, Gartzios H, Stockeld D, Granström L, Freedman J. High revision rates after laparoscopic vertical banded gastroplasty. Surg Obes Relat Dis. 2009;5(1):94–8.
13. Balsiger BM, Poggio J, Mai J, Kelly K, Sarr MG. Ten and more years after vertical banded gastroplasty as primary operation for morbid obesity. J Gastrointest Surg. 2000;4(6):598–605.
14. Gomez CA. Gastroplasty in morbid obesity. Surg Clin North Am. 1979;59(6):1113–20.
15. Gomez CA. Gastroplasty in morbid obesity: a progress report. World J Surg. 1981;5(6):823–8.
16. Wilkinson LH, Peloso OA. Gastric (reservoir) reduction for morbid obesity. Arch Surg. 1981;116(5):602–5.
17. Wilkinson LH. Reduction of gastric reservoir capacity. Am J Clin Nutr. 1980;33(2 Suppl):515–7.
18. Rudolf S. The history and role of gastric banding. Surg Obes Relat Dis. 2008;4(3):S7–S13.
19. Szinicz G, Müller L, Erhart W, Roth FX, Pointner R, Glaser K. "Reversible gastric banding" in surgical treatment of morbid obesity—results of animal experiments. Res Exp Med. 1989;189(1):55–60.
20. Kuzmak LI. A review of seven years' experience with silicone gastric banding. Obes Surg. 1991;1:403–8.
21. Belachew M, Legrand M, Vincent V. Laparoscopic placement of adjustable silicone gastric band in the treatment of morbid obesity: how to do it. Obes Surg. 1955;5:66–70.

22. Broadbent R, Tracey M, Harrington P. Laparoscopic gastric banding: a preliminary report. Obes Surg. 1993;3:63–7.
23. Mcbride CL, Kothari V. Evolution of laparoscopic adjustable gastric banding. Surg Clin North Am. 2011;91:1239–47.
24. Johnston D, Dachtler J, Sue-Ling HM. The magenstrasse and mill operation for morbid obesity. Obes Surg. 2003;13:10–6.
25. McMahon MJ. Laparoscopic sleeve gastrectomy: from magenstrasse and mill to sleeve. Proceedings supplement from the international consensus summit on sleeve gastrectomy. Bariatric Times. 2007: 3–4.
26. Marceau P, Biron S, Bourque RA. Biliopancreatic diversion with a new type of gastrectomy. Obes Surg. 1993;3:29–35.
27. Regan JP, Inabnet WB, Gagner M. Early experience with two-stage laparoscopic Roux-en-y gastric bypass as an alternative in the super-super obese patient. Obes Surg. 2003;13:861–4.
28. Gagner M, Gumbs AA, Milone L. Laparoscopic sleeve gastrectomy for the super-super-obese (body mass index >60 kg/m^2). Surg Today. 2008;38:399–403.
29. LaFave JW, Alden JF. Gastric bypass in the operative revision of the failed jejunoileal bypass. Arch Surg. 1979;114(4):438–44.
30. Scopinaro N, Gianetta E, Civalleri D. Bilio-pancreatic by-pass for obesity: II. Initial experience in man. Br J Surg. 1979;66:619–20.
31. Scopinaro N, Adami G, Marinari G. Biliopancreatic diversion. World J Surg. 1988;22:936–46.
32. Scopinaro N, Gianetta E, Civalleri D, Bonalumi U, Bachi V. Bilio-pancreatic bypass for obesity: II. Initial experience in man. Br J Surg. 1979;66(9):618–20.
33. Scopinaro N, Adami GF, Marinari GM, Gianetta E, Traverso E, Friedman D, Camerini G, Baschieri G, Simonelli A. Biliopancreatic diversion. World J Surg. 1998;22:936–46.
34. Scopinaro N, Gianetta E, Adami GF, Friedman D, Traverso E, Marinari GM, Cuneo S, Vitale B, Ballari F, Colombini M, Baschieri G, Bachi V. Biliopancreatic diversion for obesity at eighteen years. Surgery. 1996;119(3):261–8.
35. Scopinaro N. Biliopancreatic diversion: mechanisms of action and long-term results. Obes Surg. 2006;16:683–9.
36. Ito C, Mason EE, Besten LD. Experimental studies on gastric bypass versus standard ulcer operations. Tohoku J Exp Med. 1969;97(3):269–77.
37. Alden JF. Gastric and jejunoileal bypass: a comparison in the treatment of morbid obesity. Arch Surg. 1977;112(7):799–806.
38. Phillips BT, Shikora SA. The history of metabolic and bariatric surgery: development of standards for patient safety and efficacy. Metabolism. 2018;79:97–107.
39. Wittgrove AC, Clark GW, Tremblay LJ. Laparoscopic gastric bypass, Roux-en-Y: preliminary report of five cases. Obes Surg. 1994;4(4):353–7.
40. Griffen WO Jr, Young VL, Stevenson CC. A prospective comparison of gastric and jejunoileal bypass procedures for morbid obesity. Surg Obes Relat Dis. 2005;1(2):163–72.

Chapter 3
Physiology of Obesity and Obesity Related Diseases

Sneha Mishra and Natasha A. Sioda

Coronary Heart Disease

The physiology of obesity and coronary heart disease (CHD) involves a complex interplay between metabolic, hormonal, and inflammatory processes.

- Adipose Tissue Dysfunction:
  - In obesity, excess fat, particularly visceral fat, leads to adipose tissue dysfunction.
  - Adipocytes in visceral fat secrete inflammatory cytokines (e.g., TNF-α, IL-6) and non-esterified fatty acids (NEFAs), which promote systemic inflammation and metabolic disturbances.
- Insulin Resistance
  - Obesity, especially abdominal obesity, is strongly linked to insulin resistance.
  - Visceral fat releases NEFAs directly into the portal circulation, impairing the liver's ability to regulate glucose and lipid metabolism. This leads to hyperglycemia and hyperlipidemia, both risk factors for CHD [1].
- Inflammation
  - Obesity triggers chronic low-grade inflammation through the release of pro-inflammatory molecules from fat tissue.
  - This inflammation contributes to endothelial dysfunction, plaque formation, and arterial stiffening, all of which increase the risk of CHD [2].

S. Mishra · N. A. Sioda (✉)
Mayo Clinic, Phoenix, AZ, USA
e-mail: mishra.sneha@mayo.edu; sioda.natasha@mayo.edu

© The Author(s), under exclusive license to Springer Nature Switzerland AG 2025
J. A. Madura II et al. (eds.), *Bariatric Surgery Clerkship*, Contemporary Surgical Clerkships, https://doi.org/10.1007/978-3-031-92964-9_3

- Abnormal Fat Distribution
    - Central or abdominal obesity is particularly harmful, as visceral fat is more metabolically active and directly affects hepatic and cardiovascular health.
    - Waist circumference and waist-to-hip ratio are stronger predictors of CHD risk than BMI [3].
- Endothelial Dysfunction
    - The metabolic disturbances caused by obesity impair endothelial function, reducing the production of nitric oxide, which is essential for blood vessel dilation.
    - This promotes atherosclerosis and increases the risk of heart attacks and strokes.
- Increased Cardiac Workload
    - Obesity leads to a hyperdynamic circulatory state, where the heart works harder to meet the metabolic demands of excess adipose tissue and increased fat-free mass [4].
- Left Ventricular Hypertrophy (LVH)
    - Increased afterload from obesity-induced hypertension and elevated cardiac output causes eccentric and concentric LV hypertrophy, contributing to heart failure [4].
- Diastolic Dysfunction
    - Obesity impairs diastolic function, which can progress to heart failure. Fat infiltration in the heart muscle, also known as "fatty heart," can disrupt normal conduction and muscle function.

Obesity-Related Pathophysiology in Atrial Fibrillation [5]

- Inflammation
    - EAT releases IL-6, TNF-α, and NLRP3 inflammasome cytokines, driving fibrosis and oxidative stress.
- Fibrosis
    - Profibrotic factors (e.g., TGF-β, cadherin-11) from EAT promote atrial fibrosis and structural remodeling.
- Oxidative Stress
    - Obesity-induced ROS production impairs autophagy and remodels ion channels.

- Autonomic Dysfunction
  - Increased sympathetic/vagal activity shortens ERP, promoting arrhythmias.
- Electrical Remodeling
  - Fat infiltration and altered ion channels (e.g., reduced sodium/calcium currents) disrupt conduction.
- Calcium Dysregulation
  - TNF-α reduces SERCA2A, causing delayed afterdepolarizations and arrhythmogenesis.
- RAAS Activation
  - EAT-derived angiotensin II promotes fibrosis and remodeling.
- EAT Expansion: Increased EAT volume contributes to atrial enlargement, fibrosis, and electrical abnormalities.

Hypertension

This passage explores the complex mechanisms behind obesity-induced hypertension. It highlights multiple factors contributing to the condition including:

- Hemodynamic Alterations: Obesity leads to changes in vascular tone, with central obesity associated with higher systemic vascular resistance (SVR) and lower cardiac output (CO), while peripheral obesity shows the opposite.
- Endothelial Dysfunction: Adipose tissue secretes various adipokines (like angiotensinogen, angiotensin II, aldosterone) which can impair endothelial function. In obesity, these adipokines cause vascular constriction and increase plasma renin activity, further contributing to hypertension.
- Structural Changes: The endothelial glycocalyx, a protective layer, becomes thinner and stiffer with obesity, reducing the function of key ion channels responsible for vasodilation.
- Oxidative Stress: Excess free fatty acids (FFAs) increase reactive oxygen species (ROS) production, leading to vascular injury and contributing to hypertension. FFAs also activate NADPH oxidase, which exacerbates ROS production and stimulates the sympathetic nervous system.
- Renal Injury
  - Increased visceral fat compresses the kidneys, impairing kidney function, and activating the renin-angiotensin system. This causes increased sodium reabsorption, leading to elevated blood pressure.

- Hyperinsulinemia and Insulin Resistance
  - These are common in obesity and increase blood pressure by activating the renin-angiotensin system, enhancing sympathetic nervous system activity, and increasing sodium reabsorption in the kidneys.
- Sleep Apnea
  - Highly prevalent in obese individuals, sleep apnea contributes to hypertension via neurohormonal dysregulation, inflammation, and elevated endothelin levels due to hypoxia.
- Leptin-Melanocortin Pathway
  - Leptin, secreted by adipose tissue, signals fat storage to the brain and affects sympathetic nervous system activity, increasing blood pressure through sodium retention and renin-angiotensin system activation [6].
  - Each of these factors acts simultaneously, creating a multifaceted pathophysiology for obesity-related hypertension.

Hyperlipidemia

- Impaired Fat Metabolism
  - Obesity leads to impaired adipocyte function, with reduced fatty acid trapping and excessive lipolysis, resulting in high circulating nonesterified fatty acids (NEFAs).
- Atherogenic Dyslipidemia
  - This condition is characterized by elevated triglycerides, increased levels of small dense low-density lipoprotein (sdLDL) particles, and reduced high-density lipoprotein (HDL) levels, all contributing to a higher risk of atherosclerosis and CHD.
- Low HDL Levels
  - Obesity-related insulin resistance reduces lipoprotein lipase activity and enhances cholesteryl ester transfer protein (CETP)-mediated lipid exchange, leading to lower HDL levels. Reduced adiponectin levels may also contribute to this.

Metabolic Dysfunction-Associated Steatotic Liver Disease (MASLD)

- Visceral adiposity

  - Obesity, particularly central obesity, leads to excessive visceral fat accumulation, which is strongly linked to insulin resistance and liver fat accumulation.

- Inflammatory cytokines

  - Visceral fat produces pro-inflammatory cytokines like TNF-α, IL-6, and IL-1β, which promote systemic and hepatic inflammation, worsening insulin resistance.

- Reduced adiponectin

  - Obesity decreases levels of adiponectin, an anti-inflammatory hormone that improves insulin sensitivity, contributing to metabolic dysfunction in MASLD.

- Increased free fatty acids (FFAs)

  - Excess visceral fat releases FFAs into circulation, leading to increased liver fat deposition and triglyceride accumulation.

- Lipolysis dysregulation

  - In obesity, hormone-sensitive lipase (HSL) activity increases, breaking down triglycerides into FFAs that accumulate in the liver, promoting steatosis.

- Mitochondrial dysfunction

  - Obesity-induced insulin resistance reduces fatty acid oxidation in mitochondria, leading to fat buildup and oxidative stress in the liver.

- Altered lipid metabolism

  - Obesity increases hepatic production of VLDL (very-low-density lipoproteins), particularly VLDL1, contributing to fat accumulation and liver damage.

- Oxidative stress

  - Obesity accelerates reactive oxygen species (ROS) production due to abnormal lipid metabolism, further damaging liver cells and promoting MASLD progression [7]

Type 2 Diabetes Mellitus

- Insulin Resistance
  - Pancreatic Beta cells are responsible for the secretion of insulin into the portal vein which is delivered to the liver.
  - The liver is responsible for the majority of insulin clearance in the body.
  - The overall function of pancreatic B-cells is correlated to whether patients develop type 2 diabetes mellitus.
  - Elevated levels of FFA concentrations are seen in patients with obesity and negatively impact Beta-cells.
  - Obesity also leads to complex changes in adipose tissue metabolism leading to insulin resistance [8].

References

1. Romero-Corral A, Montori VM, Somers VK, Korinek J, Thomas RJ, Allison TG, et al. Association of bodyweight with total mortality and with cardiovascular events in coronary artery disease: a systematic review of cohort studies. Lancet. 2006;368(9536):666–78.
2. Tousoulis D, Antoniades C, Stefanadis C. Assessing inflammatory status in cardiovascular disease. Heart. 2007;93(8):1001–7.
3. Yusuf S, Hawken S, Ounpuu S, Dans T, Avezum A, Lanas F, et al. Effect of potentially modifiable risk factors associated with myocardial infarction in 52 countries (the INTERHEART study): case-control study. Lancet. 2004;364(9438):937–52.
4. Vasan RS. Cardiac function and obesity. Heart. 2003;89(10):1127–9.
5. Rina S, Olivia B, Abbie H, Katie T, Manish K, Holmes A, et al. Impact of obesity on atrial fibrillation pathogenesis and treatment options. J Am Heart Assoc. 2023;13(1):e032277.
6. El Meouchy P, Wahoud M, Allam S, Chedid R, Karam W, Karam S. Hypertension related to obesity: pathogenesis, characteristics and factors for control. Int J Mol Sci. 2022;23(20):12305.
7. Yanai H, Adachi H, Hakoshima M, Iida S, Katsuyama H. Metabolic-dysfunction-associated steatotic liver disease-its pathophysiology, association with atherosclerosis and cardiovascular disease, and treatments. Int J Mol Sci. 2023;24(20):15473.
8. Klein S, Gastaldelli A, Yki-Järvinen H, Scherer PE. Why does obesity cause diabetes? Cell Metab. 2022;34(1):11–20. https://doi.org/10.1016/j.cmet.2021.12.012. PMID: 34986330; PMCID: PMC8740746.

Chapter 4
Pre-operative Preparation for Bariatric Surgery

Natasha A. Sioda, Benjamin Veenstra, John Timothy Prior, John Raynak, and Narjeet Khurmi

The Bariatric Surgery Candidate

Natasha A. Sioda and Benjamin Veenstra

Introduction

Determining if bariatric surgery is a right fit for a patient is essential. The long-term goal of bariatric surgery includes improving medical co-morbidities, limiting peri-operative complications, and improving overall quality of life.

Weight loss following bariatric surgery has been shown to result in greater than 60% excess weight loss (%EWL) which is superior to other non-operative forms of weight loss including diet and exercise [1]. In addition to this, nearly all obesity related diseases have documented improvement following bariatric surgery which is essential when counseling your patient. There have been multiple publications and studies demonstrating the safety and efficacy of bariatric surgery in improving associated metabolic diseases and decreasing overall mortality [1].

N. A. Sioda (✉) · J. T. Prior · J. Raynak · N. Khurmi
Mayo Clinic, Phoenix, AZ, USA
e-mail: sioda.natasha@mayo.edu; prior.john@mayo.edu; raynak.john@mayo.edu; khurmi.narjeet@mayo.edu

B. Veenstra
Mayo Clinic, Jacksonville, FL, USA
e-mail: veenstra.benjamin@mayo.edu

Criteria

- In 1991, the National Institutes of Health (NIH) developed a standard criterion for selecting patients for bariatric surgery.
- The threshold for bariatric surgery included a body mass index (BMI) ≥ 40 kg/m^2 or BMI ≥ 35 kg/m^2 with comorbidities.
- In recent years, there have been updates to the recommended criteria for bariatric surgery selection.
- In 2022, the American Society for Metabolic and Bariatric Surgery (ASMBS) and International Federation for the Surgery of Obesity and Metabolic Disorders convened and published updated criteria for bariatric surgery.
- The updated criteria included:
  - Patients with a BMI of ≥ 35 kg/m^2 regardless of combormidities
  - BMI of ≥ 30 kg/m^2 with type II diabetes (T2D)
  - Patients with a BMI between 30 and 34.9 kg/m^2 that experienced difficulty in achieving sustainable and significant weight loss [1].

Asian Populations

- Asian populations experience cardiovascular disease and metabolic disease at a lower BMI compared to non-Asian populations.
- To reflect these observations, the BMI threshold for obesity in Asian populations is between 25–27.5 kg/m^2 [1].
- Asian patients experiencing obesity within this BMI threshold are considered candidates for bariatric surgery.

Age

- With regards to age, there is no set age limit on who can qualify for bariatric surgery.
- Patients should be evaluated for frailty and the morbidity risk associated with any obesity related co-morbidities which would preclude them from surgery [1, 2].
- Selected patients older than 70 years old do not have a higher rate of postoperative complications, and experience the same benefits as younger patients [3].
- For children and adolescents, the American Academy of Pediatrics and the ASMBS recommend considering bariatric surgery in patients with a BMI >120% of the 95% with major co-morbidity or a BMI of >140% of the 95% after careful evaluation from a multi-disciplinary team [1, 4].

Staged Procedures

- Weight loss after bariatric surgery has been shown to improve post-operative outcomes in other surgeries including abdominal wall hernia repair, transplant surgery, and knee arthroplasty [1].
- Because of the improved outcomes observed in these surgeries, performing bariatric surgery prior to these surgeries may provide benefit to these patients

The Bariatric Candidate

- Ultimately, determining the candidacy for bariatric surgery requires a multidisciplinary team and appropriate pre-operative counseling.

Bariatric Surgery Education and Counseling

John Timothy Prior and Benjamin Veenstra

Introduction

Patients that are interested in undergoing bariatric surgery require extensive pre-operative work up to evaluate their candidacy for surgery. They meet with a multidisciplinary team that can include a bariatric surgeon, psychologist, nutritionist, and internal medicine physician or endocrinologist.

Surgeon Assessment

- Meeting with the surgeon establishes the surgeon-patient relationship.
- It allows the surgeon to assess the patient's candidacy for surgery as discussed in the previous chapter.
- The surgeon will discuss potential surgeries including gastric banding, sleeve gastrectomy, Roux-en Y gastric bypass, and biliopancreatic diversion with duodenal switch. The details of these surgeries will be in a later chapter.
- The current two most common surgeries are sleeve gastrectomy and gastric bypass. Both surgeries have relatively similar outcomes, but gastric bypass is associated with more weight loss and improvement in obesity related comorbidities [5].

Psychologist Assessment

- The role of a psychologist is important in both the pre-operative and post-operative setting.
- Many psychologic disorders can affect a person's food intake and dietary choices.
- Overeating can be a maladaptive behavior to help cope with depression, stress, and anxiety and be a cause of obesity [6].
- Treatment of these disorders is beneficial to the patient's overall health and can improve weight loss on their own.
- Also, patients can undergo behavior modification therapy to learn how to reduce using eating as a support mechanism.

Nutritionist Assessment

- Patients will also meet with a nutritionist to learn and establish healthy eating habits.
- Poor dietary habits are a significant contributor to obesity and its related comorbidities.
- Educating patients on proper dietary choices and proving they can follow a diet is essential for the success of bariatric surgery [7].
- In addition, due to the restrictive nature of bariatric surgery, patients need counseling on how to adjust their diet to fit their restricted stomach.
- This includes steps such as not drinking anything 30 minutes before and after meals, taking small sips fluids and small bites of food, appropriate protein intake, and restricting meals to 4 oz. of food at a time.

Internal Medicine Assessment

- Bariatric patients often have comorbidities, such as diabetes mellitus, hypertension, and hyperlipidemia.
- They meet with an internal medicine doctor and/or an endocrinologist for optimization and management before surgery.
- In particular, the management of diabetes is important before surgery as patients with a high HbA1c have increased risks of wound healing [8].
- Ideally a patient's HbA1c should be below 7.0% but hospital policies may allow surgery on higher HbA1cs [9].
- In addition, other medical conditions including thyroid disorders, PCOS, and Cushing's should be addressed before bariatric surgery to improve weight loss.

Other Specialty Assessments

Other specialties may be involved preoperatively and postoperatively to optimize outcomes for bariatric patients.

Plastic Surgery
- Assist in managing excess skin after significant weight loss. These surgeries include panniculectomy and body contouring.
- The surgeries are done after patients have reached a plateau in their weight loss. They are done both to reduce infection risk as well as to improve the psychiatric components of dealing with the excess skin.

Cardiology
- May be consulted if patients have heart related comorbidities or the patient needs cardiac clearance before surgery.

Physical Therapy
- May be involved to improve patient's mobility before surgery as well as after.

Anesthesia
- Patient's may also benefit from having an appointment with anesthesia before surgery as bariatric patient often have Obstructive Sleep Apnea (OSA), can have challenging intubations, as well as physiological difficulties with inhaled gases in the obese population.

Sleep Medicine
- May be consulted as OSA is associated with higher perioperative complications and is more common in the bariatric population versus the general population [10, 11].

Laboratory Workup

- Other aspects of the pre-operative work up include labs and counseling about expectations.
- A patient should undergo extensive workup before surgery to assess their metabolic and nutritional status.
- This includes a complete blood count, complete metabolic panel, fasting blood glucose, hemoglobin A1c, lipid panel, urinalysis, coagulation studies, vitamin B12, folic acid, vitamin-D, iron studies, albumin, and prealbumin for nutritional status [12].

Patient Modifiers

Weight Loss
- While no hard-set rule for preoperative weight loss exists, studies have shown that patients who lose 5–10% of their weight before surgery have improved post op outcomes [9, 12].
- Pre-operative weight loss is associated with less complications and can decrease the size of the liver [9, 12].

Smoking Cessation
- Patients should also stop smoking before surgery [9].
- Smoking is associated with an increased risk of developing a marginal ulcer [13].

NSAID Cessation
- In addition, patients should stop taking NSAIDs due to the increased risk of developing peptic ulcers.
- Proton pump inhibitors are often prescribed after bariatric surgery to reduce the risk of developing ulcers [14].

Post-surgical Care

Nutritional Supplementation
- After surgery, patients should take vitamins, calcium, B12, and additional protein to help with healing after surgery as well as to make sure they get adequate nutrition due to the altered anatomy. Nutrition will be discussed in further detail in a later chapter.

Ursodiol
- If a patient still has their gallbladder, they may be prescribed ursodiol to reduce the risk of developing cholecystitis [15]. Indications for Ursodiol will be discussed in further detail in a later chapter.

Hypertensive and Diabetic Medication
- Patients should also follow closely with their primary care provider to adjust their antihypertensive or diabetes medications as both hypertension and diabetes improve after bariatric surgery.

Diet Progression
- Patients are started on a clear liquid diet before discharge.
- They stay on this diet for 1 week.
- They then advance to a blenderized diet for 2–4 weeks and progress to soft foods for 4–6 weeks.
- Afterwards they can have a regular diet.

Weight Loss Outcome
- Patients can expect to lose around five pounds a week after surgery for the first month. This rate of weight loss is variable.
- Patients can lose up to 80% of their excess weight (EWL) in the first year with 60% EWL the average [16].

Anesthesia Considerations in the Bariatric Patient

John Raynak and Narjeet Khurmi

Introduction

- Bariatric surgery is the current, most effective long-term treatment for morbid obesity. However, it carries significant risks due to the complex physiological conditions affecting multiple organ systems in these patients.
- Proper preoperative risk stratification is essential to identify those at the highest potential for complications. Thorough planning of anesthetic care across all three perioperative phases (pre-, intra-, and post-) is crucial to ensure patient safety during these procedures.
- In addition to standard considerations, anesthesiologists must account for altered pharmacokinetics and pharmacodynamics in this patient population, which can affect drug distribution, metabolism, and excretion [17].

Preoperative Evaluation

- Comorbidities Assessment
  - Focus on hypertension, diabetes, heart failure, obstructive sleep apnea (OSA), and obesity hypoventilation syndrome.
  - These conditions can complicate anesthetic plans and influence perioperative management [18].
  - Comprehensive evaluation and optimization before surgery is needed to minimize perioperative risk [19].
- Laboratory Evaluations
  - Essential tests: fasting blood glucose/HbA1C, lipid profiles, renal and hepatic function tests, complete blood counts, and vitamin levels.

- Assess thyroid function due to its link with obesity and effects on metabolic rate and drug metabolism [17].
- Obesity is associated with various metabolic derangements requiring thorough evaluation [18].

- Liver Function Evaluation
  - Assess for nonalcoholic fatty liver disease; significant dysfunction may require anesthetic management adjustments or contraindicate surgery [18].

- Sleep Study Indicators
  - An Apnea-Hypopnea Index (AHI) score over 30 indicates severe sleep apnea, increasing the risk of desaturation during induction.
  - Optimization of sleep apnea management is essential [17].

- OSA Management
  - Assess and optimize preoperative CPAP adherence [18].
  - Ensure CPAP therapy availability and use throughout the perioperative period to mitigate airway obstruction and hypoxia risks.

- Previous Surgical History Review
  - Important for identifying potential airway management challenges and recovery outcomes that could influence current surgical plans and/or anesthesia plans, such as induction/intubation/airway management [17].

- Contraindications for Surgery
  - Conditions such as unstable coronary artery disease, uncontrolled severe OSA, pulmonary hypertension, or poorly controlled diabetes mellitus or hypertension can preclude elective surgery.
  - Effective management may transition high-risk patients to acceptable risk categories [18].

Anesthetic Agent Selection

- Agent Selection
  - Choose agents carefully to avoid exacerbating existing or potential respiratory conditions, considering patient-specific factors, including comorbidities and drug interactions [17].
  - Adjust anesthetic dosing based on altered pharmacokinetics in obese patients [19].

- Anesthetic Dosing
  - Adjust doses of analgesics such as opioids and sedatives such as propofol and benzodiazepines to minimize respiratory depression [18].

4 Pre-operative Preparation for Bariatric Surgery

- Use total body weight (TBW) or ideal body weight (IBW) based on the drug's lipid solubility to ensure effective action [17].
- Use IBW for lipophilic drugs, such as propofol and vecuronium to avoid overdosing [18].
- Use TBW for hydrophilic drugs, such as midazolam and fentanyl, adjusting maintenance doses as necessary [17].

- Complete Neuromuscular Blockade
  - Often required for effective ventilation, especially in morbidly obese patients.
  - Use objective monitors, such as a peripheral nerve stimulator to assess for complete reversal/recovery of neuromuscular blockade to ensure adequate respiratory function postoperatively [18].

- Volatile Anesthetic Selection
  - Use agents with low blood:gas solubility, such as sevoflurane and desflurane for faster recovery and less respiratory depression [17].

- Nitrous Oxide
  - Avoid in obese patients due to increased intra-abdominal pressure risks during laparoscopic procedures [18].
  - Also important to avoid due to risk of introducing a hypoxic gas mixture in a patient population more likely to have decreased respiratory reserve, faster oxygen desaturations, and potential for right heart issues.

Airway Management

- Anatomical Challenges
  - Obese patients often have anatomically challenging airways due to short, thick necks and large tongues.
  - Prepare for difficult intubation with appropriate equipment including but not limited to intubating stylet (aka "bougie"), supraglottic airway devices (aka "LMA"), fiberoptic bronchoscopes, and tracheostomy kits.

- Positioning for Intubation
  - Use the ramped position to enhance laryngeal visibility and improve intubation success. This position elevates the patient's upper body, head and neck above chest level until the patient's tragus/external auditory meatus is in the same horizontal plane as the sternal notch.
  - The "sniffing position" aligns the oral, pharyngeal, and laryngeal axes for better laryngoscopy [18].

- Techniques for Airway Management
  - Video Laryngoscopy: Offers better glottis visualization, reducing intubation time and increasing first attempt success rates [17].

- Emergency Equipment Availability
    - Have essential tools, such as oropharyngeal airway, supraglottic airway devices (laryngeal masks), fiberoptic bronchoscopes, and tracheostomy kits ready for difficult airway situations [18].

Pulmonary Considerations

- Unique Pulmonary Challenges:
    - Obese patients often have decreased lung volumes leading to rapid oxygen desaturation with apnea.
    - Requires careful and deliberate oxygenation strategies [17].
    - Obesity-related pulmonary changes necessitate tailored ventilation strategies including maintaining peak inspiratory pressure below 35 cmH_2O and 5–7 mL/kg tidal volumes based on ideal body weight [19].
- Oxygenation Techniques:
    - Positioning: Use reverse Trendelenburg or ramped positions for preoxygenation to decrease ventilation/perfusion (V/Q) mismatch and optimize ventilation [18].
    - Preoxygenation: Use 100% oxygen with positive pressure before intubation to enhance oxygen reserves [17].
    - PEEP Maintenance: Maintain positive end-expiratory pressure during surgery to improve oxygenation and prevent atelectasis [18].
    - CPAP Utilization: Maintain home CPAP levels intraoperatively for OSA patients to ensure respiratory stability [17].

Induction of Anesthesia

- Aspiration Risk Management:
    - Consider factors, such as delayed gastric emptying in diabetic patients.
    - Morbid obesity is an independent risk factor for aspiration
    - Use prophylactic measures such as prokinetic/promotility agents and H2 receptor antagonists when necessary [18].
- Induction Techniques:
    - Use rapid sequence induction or awake fiberoptic intubation for high-risk patients.
    - Tailor approaches to the patient's risk profile and airway anatomy [17].
- Regional Anesthesia Challenges:
    - Safe and useful as part of a multimodal pain management approach.
    - Anatomical difficulties may arise due to large body habitus.

- Invasive Monitoring Requirements:
  - Additional monitoring may be needed for patients with comorbid conditions.
  - Ensure accurate blood pressure measurements and IV access; consider central access if peripheral IV is difficult [18].
  - Consider invasive blood pressure monitors (arterial line) if poorly fitting blood pressure cuff—leads to inaccurate readings
- Venous Thromboembolism Prophylaxis:
  - Implement anticoagulants and lower extremity mechanical devices to reduce thromboembolism risk [17].

Intraoperative Management

- Anesthetic Technique Selection:
  - Tailor the anesthetic technique to the patient's conditions and surgical needs.
  - Utilize Total Intravenous Anesthesia (TIVA) and/or inhalation anesthesia as appropriate.
  - The choice will depend on patient comorbidities, potential airway challenges, and the need for rapid recovery [18].
  - TIVA can reduce postoperative nausea and vomiting (PONV) and may offer better hemodynamic stability [19].
- Ventilation Strategies:
  - Use tidal volumes of 6–8 mL/kg of Ideal Body Weight (IBW) to minimize barotrauma risk and ensure adequate ventilation.
  - Obese patients may need higher PEEP, however, more research is needed on "optimal" PEEP as part of a protective ventilatory strategy that improves postoperative pulmonary outcomes [20].
  - Close monitoring of end-tidal CO_2 and oxygen saturation is essential to maintain optimal respiratory function [17].
- Positioning Importance:
  - Proper positioning prevents respiratory impairment and facilitates adequate ventilation and oxygenation.
  - Obese patients may have difficulty tolerating steep Trendelenburg positions due to increased airway pressures and reduced lung volumes created by the increased weight on the diaphragm and thorax [18].
  - The reverse Trendelenburg position can improve respiratory mechanics by reducing intra-abdominal pressure/weight on the diaphragm and thorax [19].

- Fluid Management Strategies
    - Careful fluid management is crucial to avoid complications from volume overload or dehydration.
    - Use goal-directed fluid therapy, guided by dynamic hemodynamic parameters, to optimize hemodynamic stability and improve surgical outcomes [17].
- PONV Prophylaxis
    - Implement strategies to prevent postoperative nausea and vomiting (PONV), a common concern in bariatric surgery patients.
    - Include the use of antiemetics such as ondansetron, dexamethasone, and droperidol, as well as non-pharmacological measures [18].
- Pain Management:
    - Use a multimodal approach to minimize opioid use and reduce respiratory depression risk.
    - Employ non-opioid analgesics, regional anesthesia techniques, and adjuvants like gabapentinoids [17].
- Emergence from Anesthesia:
    - Ensure complete neuromuscular blockade reversal before extubation to prevent respiratory complications.
    - Support pulmonary recovery with noninvasive ventilation techniques, especially for patients with OSA or other respiratory issues [18].

Postoperative Management

- Consistent Care Environment:
    - Post-bariatric surgery patients benefit from CPAP or bilevel positive airway pressure machines to monitor and support respiratory function, particularly those with pre-existing OSA [17].
    - Ensuring continuity of care with appropriate respiratory support can reduce postoperative hypoxemia and related complications.
- Complication Awareness:
    - Vigilant monitoring for potential complications, focusing on wound healing, gastrointestinal, pulmonary, and cardiovascular issues.
    - Laparoscopic procedures typically have lower complication rates than open surgeries, but early identification and management of complications are crucial for improving outcomes [17].
- Reoperation Considerations:
    - Review previous anesthesia records to assess risks, particularly concerning aspiration and difficult airways.

- Detailed planning and preparation can mitigate risks associated with reoperation and enhance surgical outcomes [18].

- Long-term Complications:

  - Patients may experience long-term complications such as strictures and nutritional deficiencies post-surgery.
  - Increased GERD
  - Regular follow-up and nutritional support are important to address these issues and ensure ongoing health and well-being.

Conclusion

- Comprehensive Anesthesia Management:

  - Effective management of bariatric surgery requires a thorough understanding of the unique anatomic and physiologic challenges posed by obesity.
  - Anesthesia providers must be knowledgeable and skilled in optimizing perioperative care to address these challenges effectively.

- Enhancing Patient Safety:

  - Addressing patient-specific needs throughout the perioperative period—from preoperative evaluation to postoperative care—can significantly help improve surgical outcomes and patient safety.
  - This comprehensive approach ensures effective management of obesity-related complexities, reducing complications and promoting recovery [17].

References

1. Eisenberg D, Shikora SA, Aarts E, Aminian A, Angrisani L, Cohen RV, de Luca M, Faria SL, Goodpaster KPS, Haddad A, Himpens JM, Kow L, Kurian M, Loi K, Mahawar K, Nimeri A, O'Kane M, Papasavas PK, Ponce J, Pratt JSA, Rogers AM, Steele KE, Suter M, Kothari SN. 2022 American Society of Metabolic and Bariatric Surgery (ASMBS) and International Federation for the Surgery of Obesity and Metabolic Disorders (IFSO) indications for metabolic and bariatric surgery. Obes Surg. 2023;33(1):3–14.
2. Gondal AB, Hsu CH, Zeeshan M, Hamidi M, Joseph B, Ghaderi I. A frailty index and the impact of frailty on postoperative outcomes in older patients after bariatric surgery. Surg Obes Relat Dis. 2019;9:1582–8.
3. Hammond JB, Webb CJ, Pulivarthi VSKK, Pearson DG, Harold KL, Madura JA II. Is there an upper age limit for bariatric surgery? Laparoscopic gastric bypass outcomes in septuagenarians. Obes Surg. 2020;30:2482–6.
4. Pratt JSA, Browne A, Browne NT, Bruzoni M, Cohen M, Desai A, Inge T, Linden BC, Mattar SG, Michalsky M, Podkameni D, Reichard KW, Stanford FC, Zeller MH, Zitsman J. ASMBS pediatric metabolic and bariatric surgery guidelines. Surg Obes Relat Dis. 2018;14(7):882–901.
5. Biter LU, 't Hart JWH, Noordman BJ, Smulders JF, Nienhuijs S, Dunkelgrün M, et al. Long-term effect of sleeve gastrectomy vs Roux-en-Y gastric bypass in people living with severe

obesity: a phase III multicentre randomised controlled trial (SleeveBypass). Lancet Reg Health Eur. 2024;38:100836.
6. Snyder AG. Psychological assessment of the patient undergoing bariatric surgery. Ochsner J. 2009;9(3):144–8.
7. Schlottmann F, Nayyar A, Herbella FAM, Patti MG. Preoperative evaluation in bariatric surgery. J Laparoendosc Adv Surg Tech A. 2018;28(8):925–9.
8. Christman AL, Selvin E, Margolis DJ, Lazarus GS, Garza LA. Hemoglobin A1c predicts healing rate in diabetic wounds. J Invest Dermatol. 2011;131(10):2121–7.
9. Mechanick JI, Youdim A, Jones DB, Garvey WT, Hurley DL, McMahon MM, et al. Clinical practice guidelines for the perioperative nutritional, metabolic, and nonsurgical support of the bariatric surgery patient—2013 update: cosponsored by American Association of Clinical Endocrinologists, The Obesity Society, and American Society for Metabolic & Bariatric Surgery. Obesity. 2013;21(S1):S1–27.
10. Opperer M, Cozowicz C, Bugada D, Mokhlesi B, Kaw R, Auckley D, et al. Does obstructive sleep apnea influence perioperative outcome? A qualitative systematic review for the Society of Anesthesia and Sleep Medicine Task Force on Preoperative Preparation of Patients with Sleep-Disordered Breathing. Anesth Analg. 2016;122(5):1321–34.
11. Kapur VK, Auckley DH, Chowdhuri S, Kuhlmann DC, Mehra R, Ramar K, et al. Clinical practice guideline for diagnostic testing for adult obstructive sleep apnea: an American Academy of Sleep Medicine clinical practice guideline. J Clin Sleep Med. 2017;13(3):479–504.
12. Mechanick JI, Youdim A, Jones DB, Timothy Garvey W, Hurley DL, Molly McMahon M, et al. Clinical practice guidelines for the perioperative nutritional, metabolic, and nonsurgical support of the bariatric surgery patient—2013 update: cosponsored by American Association of Clinical Endocrinologists, The Obesity Society, and American Society for Metabolic & Bariatric Surgery. Surg Obes Relat Dis. 2013;9(2):159–91.
13. van Wissen J, Bakker N, Doodeman HJ, Jansma EP, Bonjer HJ, Houdijk AP. Preoperative methods to reduce liver volume in bariatric surgery: a systematic review. Obes Surg. 2016;26(2):251–6.
14. Giannopoulos S, Athanasiadis DI, Clapp B, Lyo V, Ghanem O, Puzziferri N, et al. Proton pump inhibitor prophylaxis after Roux-en-Y gastric bypass: a national survey of surgeon practices. Surg Obes Relat Dis. 2023;19(4):303–8.
15. Coogan AC, Williams MD, Krishnan V, Skertich NJ, Becerra AZ, Sarran M, et al. Ursodiol prescriptions following bariatric surgery: national prescribing trends and outcomes. Obes Surg. 2023;33(8):2361–7.
16. Wittgrove AC, Clark GW. Laparoscopic gastric bypass, Roux-en-Y-500 patients: technique and results, with 3-60 month follow-up. Obes Surg. 2000;10(3):233–9.
17. Gropper MA, et al. Miller's anesthesia. Philadelphia: Elsevier; 2024. p. 1124–235.
18. Cullen BF, et al. Barash, Cullen, and Stoelting's clinical anesthesia. Philadelphia: Wolters Kluwer; 2024. p. 945–85.
19. Seyni-Boureima R, et al. Challenges in anesthetic management of obese patients: a review. J Anesth Clin Res. 2022;22:98.
20. Fernandez-Bustamante A, Sprung J. Intraoperative positive end-expiratory pressure for obese patients: a step forward, a long road still ahead. Anesthesiology. 2021;134(6):838–40.

Chapter 5
Bariatric Technique and Outcomes

Nisha Rehman, David G. Pearson, Sinong Qian, Nicholas Nolan, Holly Grossman, and Natasha A. Sioda

Adjustable Gastric Banding Procedure (AGB)

Nisha Rehman and David G. Pearson

Introduction

- In the 1970s, the nonadjustable gastric band procedure was introduced with poor outcomes, however, when the first adjustable gastric band (AGB) was introduced in the 1980s results showed promising weight loss with minimal complications.
- In the 1990s, the first laparoscopically placed adjustable gastric band (LAGB) was introduced and became a popular bariatric surgery option.
- The LAGB was approved to be offered to patients in the United States in 2001. However, in 2008 when sleeve gastrectomy was introduced, the popularity of AGB began to decline, and by 2022 AGB composed only 1–2% of bariatric surgeries performed in the US [1–3].
- The main advantage of AGB is individualized adjustability and significantly lower initial operative morbidity and mortality. AGB is the placement of a restrictive inflatable balloon device 1 cm below the gastroesophageal junction around

the gastric cardia. The balloon is connected to a subcutaneous port via a tube. Saline injected into the port causes balloon inflation, narrowing the stomach at the balloon level. Therefore, the AGB reduces the size of the stomach and restricts the amount of food a person can consume [4].

Contraindications

Absolute Contraindications
- Inability to tolerate general anesthesia, uncontrollable coagulopathy

Relative Contraindications
- Cirrhosis with portal hypertension, pregnancy, Prader-Willi syndrome, malignant hyperphagia, untreated psychiatric illness, pregnancy, autoimmune connective tissue disorders, chronic inflammatory conditions, chronic corticosteroid use [1, 5]

Advantages and Disadvantages

Advantages
- Avoids risks of gastrointestinal manipulation (stapling and anastomosis)
- Completely reversible
- Technically easy
- Less morbid

Disadvantages
- Continued medical follow up for band adjustments
- Unsatisfactory weight loss
- Need for reoperation for malpositioning
- Esophageal Dysfunction [6]

Surgical Technique

Patient Positioning and Trocar Placement
- Patient placed in supine position and slight Trendelenburg position.
- For a laparoscopic approach, a 5 mm trocar is placed for camera, 15 mm working trocar, 1–2 5 mm additional working trocars, and a liver retractor are placed.

Diaphragmatic Hiatus Assessment
- At the angle of His, the peritoneum is divided via Harmonic to create an opening in the peritoneum between the angle of His and the top of the spleen

Fig. 5.1 Depiction of anatomy of stomach and Angle of HIS

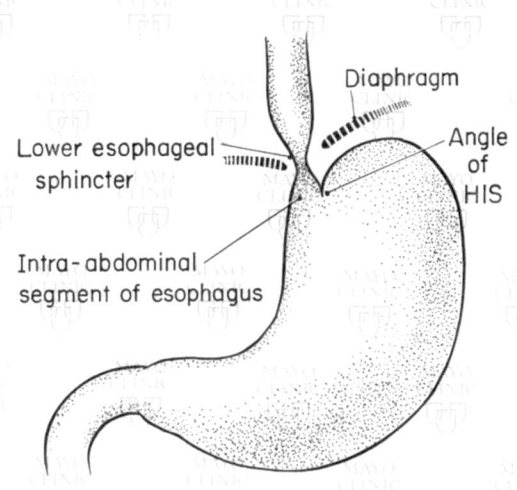

- The right crus of the diaphragm is identified.
- Any crural defects or hiatal hernias are repaired (Fig. 5.1).

Tunnel Creation
- The pars flaccida is exposed and divided.
- Using a 5 mm laparoscopic dissector, an avascular tunnel is created underneath the stomach superior to lesser sac. The tip of the dissector is angled towards the angle of His near the top of the spleen.

Gastric Band Placement
- The balloon on the device is completely deflated
- The device is inserted into the abdomen through the 15 mm trocar.
- The distal portion of the device is grabbed with the tunneling dissector at the angle of His and then pulled through the tunnel.
- The gastric band is then locked anteriorly (Fig. 5.2)

Gastro-gastric Plication
- The anterior gastric wall is plicated over the band with 3–4 interrupted, nonabsorbable sutures. This secures the distal fundus of the stomach to the gastric pouch.
- The buckle should not be covered and rotated to the right

Access Port Placement
- The tubing leading from the band is pulled through the 15 mm trocar site in the right upper quadrant.
- The access port is connected to the tubing
- The access port is secured to the fascia via four nonabsorbable sutures [1, 4, 7]

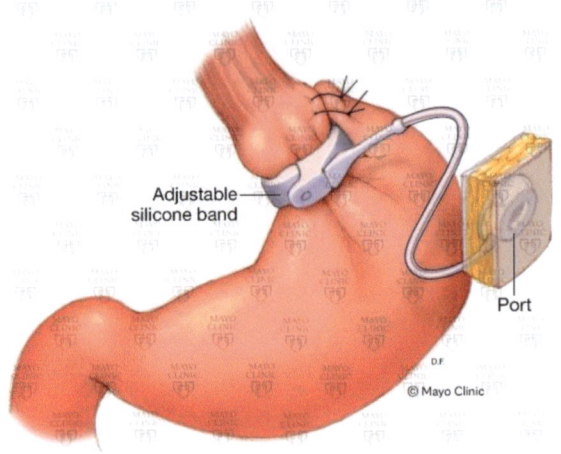

Fig. 5.2 Depiction of adjustable gastric band

Postoperative Care

- Postoperative Day 0:
  - Patients are admitted to the hospital and put on a clear liquid diet.
  - The band is not initially insufflated with saline.
- Postoperative Day 1:
  - Patients advanced to full liquids or pureed food and usually discharged.
- 4–6 weeks postoperatively:
  - Patients advanced to solid food
  - First band adjustment is usually offered under fluoroscopic guidance.
  - Saline is added in 1.0- to 1.5-mL increments to produce a desired weight loss of 1–2 kg/week.
  - Patients need to be able to swallow water before leaving the office.
  - Subsequent monthly appointments
- 2nd postoperative year:
  - The patient should be seen 2–3 times for adjustments [1].

Outcomes

Weight Loss
- Occurs gradually
- 35% excess body weight loss by 6 months

- 40% by 12 months
- 50% by 24 months
- This weight loss remains stable after 3–8 years
- 25% of patients fail to lose 50% of their excess body weight by 5 years
- Comorbid Conditions
  - Improves Type 2 Diabetes in 90% of patients
  - Resolves GERD symptoms in 80–90% of patients by 12 months
  - Improves obstructive sleep apnea in 2–33% of patients [1, 7]

Post Operative Complications

LAGB has the lowest mortality of all the bariatric procedures with an approximate 0.02% to 0.1% overall mortality, 3% 30-day morbidity, and 12% rate of late complications

Early Complications
- Deep Vein Thrombosis
- Esophageal or gastric perforation
- Esophagogastric obstruction

Late Complications
- Gastric prolapse, or a "slipped band,"
- Lower stomach herniating superiorly through the device
- Can lead to acute strangulation of the stomach
- Symptom: sudden-onset food intolerance or reflux symptoms
- Diagnosis: plain abdominal radiograph and upper GI study
- Treatment: initial deflation of the band with eventual reoperation
- Band Erosion
  - Band erodes into the stomach wall
  - Symptoms: delayed port site infections, abdominal pain, failure to suppress appetite
  - Diagnosis: Endoscopy
  - Treatment: reoperation with removal of band, repair of gastric wall and drainage
- Device Malfunction:
  - Device leaks, tube kinking, port puncture, band puncture, port dislodgement
- Band Obstruction
  - Secondary to overinflated band, low band placement, or missed hiatal hernia
  - Can lead to gastric pouch and esophageal dilation, esophagitis, esophageal dysmotility, megaesophagus, or pseudo-achalasia
  - Diagnosis: Upper GI study
  - Treatment: Deflate the band, with potential for reoperation [1, 8]

Sleeve Gastrectomy

Sinong Qian and David G. Pearson

Introduction

Sleeve gastrectomy creates a tubular, sleeve-shaped stomach by resection of the greater curvature of the gastric body and fundus. It was initially performed in 1990s as the first stage of biliopancreatic diversion with duodenal switch [9]. It has become the most frequently performed bariatric surgery in the United States since 2013 given it's technically easier comparing to other weight-loss surgeries [10].

Contraindications

- Relative contraindications include Barrett's esophagus, paraesophageal hernia, and severe gastroesophageal reflux disease [11].

Surgical Technique

Patient Positioning and Trocar Placement
- Patient is positioned supine with or without legs spread according to the surgeon's preference.
- Port placement for laparoscopic sleeve gastrectomy (Fig. 5.3): 12–15 mm port in the right mid abdomen for stapler, 10 mm periumbilical port for camera, two 5 mm working ports in the left mid and lateral abdomen, liver retractor in the subxiphoid area.
- Port placement for robotic sleeve gastrectomy (Fig. 5.4): 12 mm port in the right lateral abdomen for stapler, three 8 mm ports in right mid abdomen, left mid abdomen and left lateral abdomen for robotic instruments.

Mobilization of the Stomach
- Dissection begins by dividing the gastroepiploic arcade and opening the lesser sac approximately 5–6 cm proximal to the pylorus. Then the dissection is carried out along the greater curvature up to the highest short gastric vessels.
- Divide the gastrophrenic ligament and mobilize the angle of His from the left crus of the diaphragm.
- The stomach is then lifted to expose its posterior aspect and all posterior attachments to the stomach are freed.

Fig. 5.3 Laparoscopic sleeve gastrectomy port

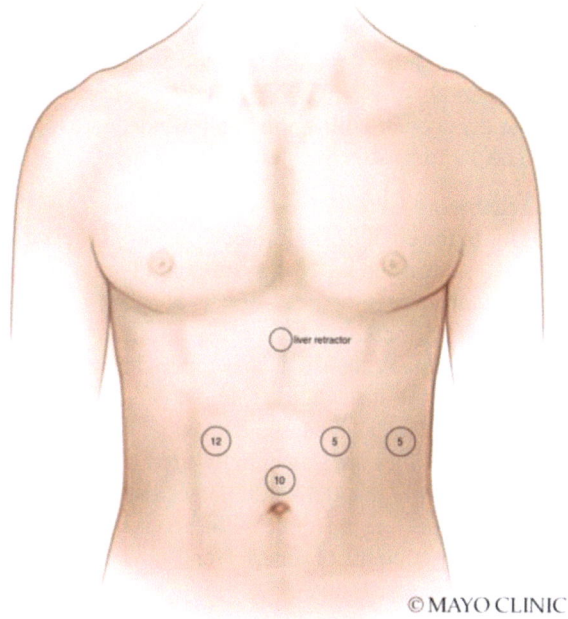

Fig. 5.4 Robotic sleeve gastrectomy port

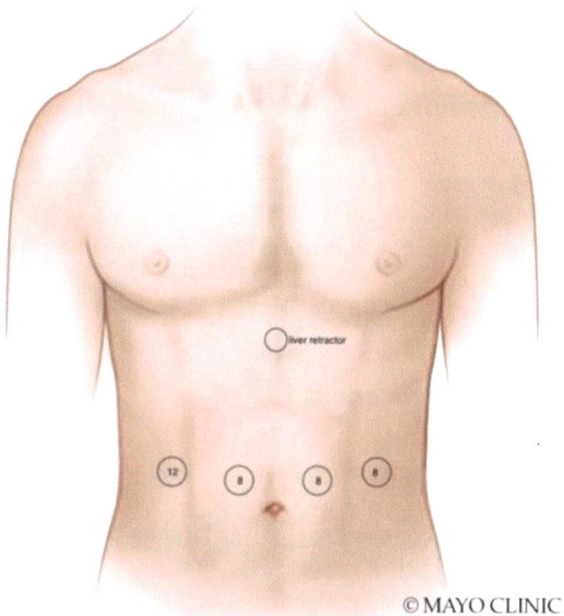

- After exposing the left crus of the diaphragm, the surgery should determine if a hiatal hernia is present. If so, a formal closure of the hiatus is mandatory since GERD and other complications are associated with its presence in the postoperative period.
- The complete mobilization to allow adequate resection of the fundus is believed to be a critical step of sleeve gastrectomy.

Gastric Sleeve Creation
- Prior to the creation of the sleeve, a 34–40 French bougie is inserted through the mouth, down the lesser curvature and the tip is placed in the prepyloric area of the stomach.
- After confirmation that no other intragastric tubes, e.g. orogastric tubes, temperature probes, the stomach is transected approximately 5–6 cm proximal to the pylorus along the bougie. Care should be taken not to divide the stomach too close to the incisura angularis to avoid stenosis at the level.
- The staple lines are sequentially fired along the bougie toward the angle of His with an angle parallel to the lesser curvature and divide the fundus 0.5–1 cm lateral to the GE junction. With each staple fire, the surgeon needs to make sure that equal amount of anterior and posterior gastric wall are resected to avoid "spiraling" of the sleeve.
- The resected portion of the stomach is then removed from the 12–15 mm port.

Leak Test
- Leak test can either performed with EGD or OG tube by insufflating the gastric sleeve with air.

Postoperative Care

- Most patients are discharged on a liquid diet on postoperative day 1 and a proton pump inhibitor for 6–8 weeks.
- Some centers will perform upper GI series with contrast on POD 1 prior to starting a diet.

Early Complications

- The most feared complication is leak.
- The incidence of leak after laparoscopic sleeve gastrectomy is 1–2%.
- The most common site for leak is along the staple line immediately below the GE junction [12].
- Patient may be asymptomatic but elevated heart rate may be the first sign.

Late Complications
- GERD
- Weight regain
- Vitamin deficiency
- Possible esophageal dysmotility

Outcomes

- The average excess weight loss after 5 years is around 60%.
- Resolution of comorbidities is excellent, around 60% for diabetes and 50% for hypertension after 5 years [13].

Gastric Bypass

Nicholas Nolan and David G. Pearson

Introduction

Gastric bypass is another form of weight loss surgery which involves creating a small gastric pouch with reconfiguration of the GI anatomy with creation of a gastrojejunostomy and a jejunojejunostomy in the classic Roux-en-Y fashion. It was first developed in the late 1970s and was later adapted to a laparoscopic surgery in the mid 1990s [14]. This procedure is defined as both a restrictive and malabsorptive.

Indications

- Preferred weight loss surgery in the setting of significant gastroesophageal reflex disease [15]

Surgical Technique

Patient Positioning and Trocar Placement
- Supine position, arms tucked

- Establish pneumoperitoneum with port placement: 12-mm in the right and left midabdomen, 5 mm ports in the left subcostal and left lateral abdomen, 10 mm port in the right periumbilical region, liver retractor placed in the subxiphoid region

Roux Limb and Jejunostomy Creation
- Using harmonic shears, the greater omentum is split allowing room for the future antecolic, antegastric roux limb creation.
- Formation of Roux Limb and jejunojejunostomy.
- To create the Roux limb, the Ligament of Treitz is first identified. The proximal jejunum is then ran 40 cm distal and is transected using a linear Endo-GIA stapler. A 75–100 cm Roux limb is then measured out. An intracorporeal jejunojejunostomy is then created with the linear Endo-GIA stapler in a side-side fashion. The mesenteric defect is then closed with running non-absorbable suture to prevent future internal herniation.

Gastric Pouch
- Then, an approximately 15–30 mL gastric pouch is created. The gastrophrenic and crural attachments are freed from the stomach. Just distal to the left gastric artery, staplers are fired sequentially with progression towards the angle of His to complete the gastric pouch. Care is taken to exclude the gastric fundus.

Creation of Gastrojejunostomy
- The roux limb is brought up in an antecolic, antegastric fashion. A back row of absorbable sutures are placed between the stomach and proximal roux limb. A gastrotomy and jejunotomy are created using electrocautery and a linear Endo-GIA is used to create the gastrojejunostomy.
- At this point, intraoperative EGD is performed and the endoscope is advance into the roux limb. The gastrojejunostomy is then closed in two layers using absorbable suture over the endoscope to ensure patency.

Leak Test
- Finally, a leak test is done with the gastrojejunostomy submerged in saline and tested with insufflation from the endoscope. Once there is confirmed to be no evidence of leak, the endoscope is carefully withdrawn and the anastomosis is examined for hemostasis

Closure of Petersons Defect
- Peterson's space is the site of potential internal herniation between the mesentery of the Roux limb and transverse mesocolon in a patient with a retrocolic roux limb. This is optionally closed based on surgeon preference.

Postoperative Considerations
- Proton Pump Inhibitors should be used for at least the first 30 days to prevent early marginal ulceration
- Initially, transition all oral medication to Elixir/crushed form and avoid extended release medications

- Calcium, Iron, Vitamin D, and Vitamin B12 supplementation are recommended to prevent deficiencies
- In patients who have not undergone cholecystectomy, Ursodiol for 6–12 months can be used to help decrease the risk of gallstone formation in the setting of rapid weight loss
- Patients are usually discharged on postoperative day 1–2 on a bariatric clear liquid diet (Fig. 5.5)

Complications
- Early complications: Early bowel obstruction, anastomotic leak/bleed, DVT/PE, dumping syndrome
- Late complications: Bowel obstruction, internal hernia, gastro-gastric fistula, vitamin deficiency, marginal ulceration, weight regain

Outcomes
- Expected percent of excess weight loss is estimated to be between 52 and 69% [16–19]
- Approximate −15 reduction in BMI
- Resolution or improvement in medical comorbidities:
    - Diabetes: 62–83%
    - Hypertension: 38–79%
    - Dyslipidemia: 53–71%
    - OSA: 66%
- Mortality rate 0.1–0.5%

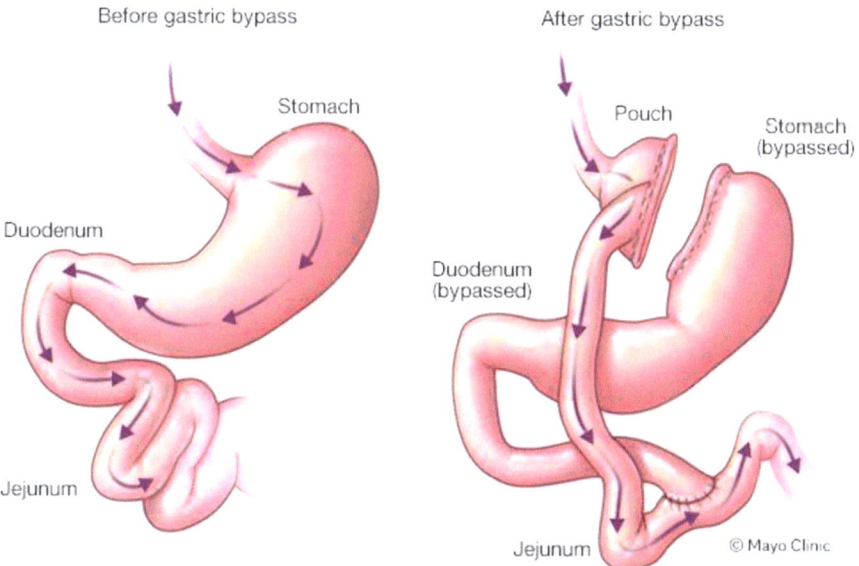

Fig. 5.5 Anatomy of gastric bypass

Biliopancreatic Diversion

Holly Grossman and David G. Pearson

Introduction

Biliopancreatic diversion (BPD) was originally described by Scopinaro in 1979 as an alternative to jejunoileal bypass [20], which included:

- Distal gastrectomy, gastrojejunostomy, and jejunojejunostomy
- Common channel length of 50 cm
- Alimentary limb length of 250 cm

Later, the duodenal switch (DS) was described by DeMeester in 1987 to improve marginal ulceration and gastritis [21], which included:

- Common channel length of 100 cm
- Longitudinal gastrectomy

These procedures were then combined to create the modern BPD-DS by Hess & Hess in 1998 [22].

Anatomy

Duodenal switch entails a sleeve gastrectomy combined with a duodenoenterostomy (Fig. 5.6).
  Basic components of biliopancreatic diversion with duodenal switch (BPD-DS):

- Longitudinal gastrectomy for calorie restriction and decreased acid production
- Alimentary limb of approximately 250 cm to decrease caloric absorption
- Longer common channel of approximately 100 cm to allow mixing of food with bile and pancreatic enzymes from the alimentary and biliary limb

Contraindications

Similar to contraindications for other bariatric surgeries, including:

- Untreated psychiatric or eating disorders
- Severe liver disease
- Noncompliance with follow up
- Previous jejunoileal bypass or malnutrition

Fig. 5.6 Anatomic layout of duodenal switch

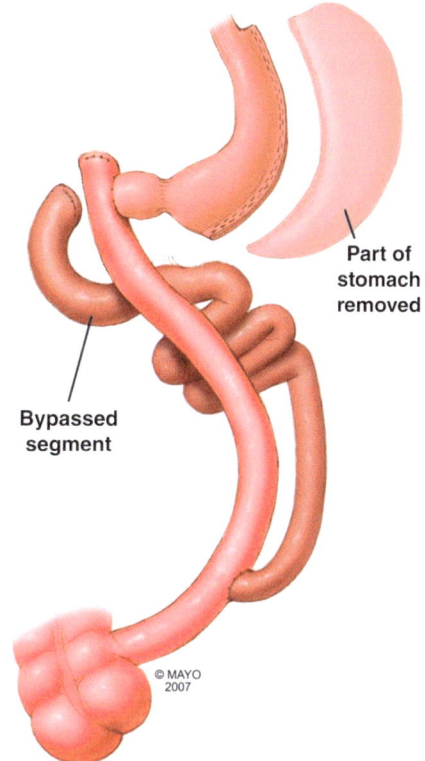

As it includes a sleeve gastrectomy, it is relatively contraindicated in patients with:

- Barrett's Esophagus
- Paraesophageal hernia
- Gastric reflux (Fig. 5.7)

Advantages and Disadvantages

Advantages
- Duodenal switch differs from traditional BPD in that it maintains the lesser curvature of the stomach
- In addition, it preserves the pylorus and first portion of the duodenum, which:
  - Helps limit marginal ulceration
  - Decreases incidence of dumping syndrome
- Provides a combination of restriction and malabsorption
- No isolated stomach as the excluded stomach is removed, which differs from traditional Roux-en-Y bypass

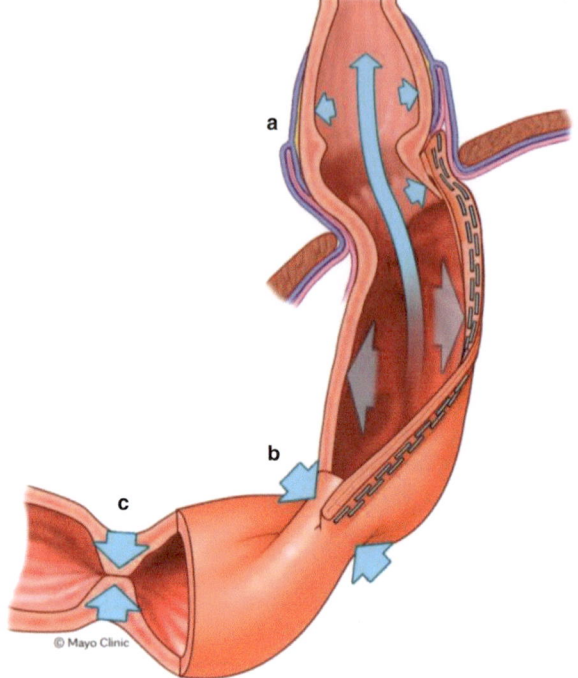

Fig. 5.7 Worsening of gastric reflux following sleeve gastrectomy from: (**a**) disruption of the lower esophageal sphincter; (**b**) angulation, and (**c**) pylorospasm

- Does not introduce a foreign body, as is seen with gastric banding
- A conversion option for unsuccessful Roux-en-Y bypass and gastric sleeve [23] (Fig. 5.8)
- Effective option for more obese patients (BMI >50)

Disadvantages
- More technically difficult than other bariatric procedures with a steep learning curve that typically limits its use outside of specialized centers [25]
- Requires long-term follow-up for malabsorption
    - Jejunal exclusion: iron and vitamin B12 malabsorption
    - Fat soluble vitamin deficiencies [26]

Surgical Approach

Laparoscopic Versus Open
- Similar to other procedures, the laparoscopic approach requires a longer overall operative time
- Allows for a shorter hospital stay and improved postoperative pain levels when compared to open procedures
- It has also shown similar complication rates at 30 days when compared to open procedures [27]

5 Bariatric Technique and Outcomes

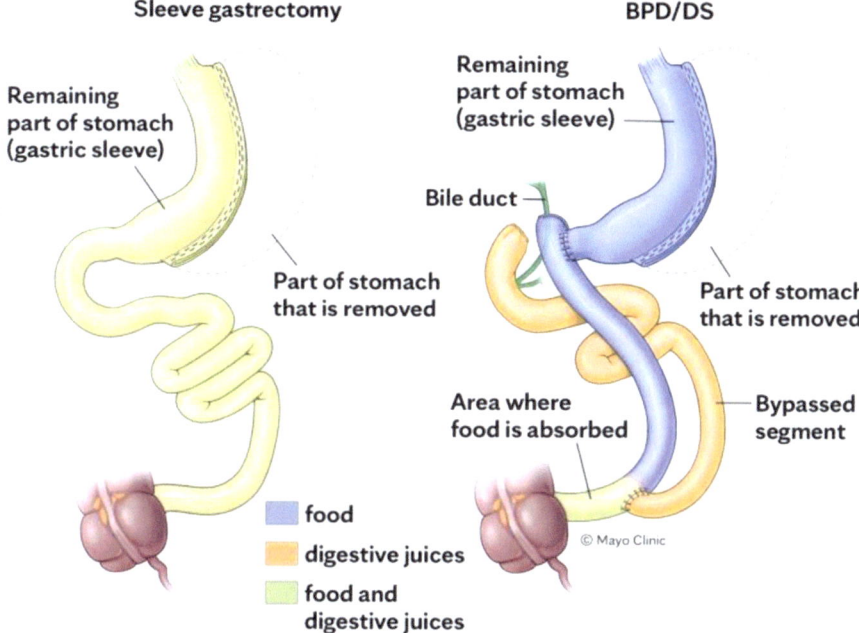

Fig. 5.8 Comparison of sleeve gastrectomy and duodenal switch

Robotic
- Robotic approaches for BPD-DS can be beneficial due to technical complexity of the case and can reduce the need for intraoperative assistance
- However, it does require longer operative times and may be associated with a higher risk of thromboembolism [28]

Surgical Technique

Gastric Mobilization
- Using a vessel sealing device, open the gastrocolic ligament which attaches the greater curvature to the transverse colon

Short Gastric Vessel Ligation
- Ligate short gastric vessels along the greater curvature of the stomach, starting approximately 6 cm from the pylorus

Vertical Sleeve Gastrectomy
- Using a linear stapler, create vertical sleeve gastrectomy
- Stapling starts approximately 2–6 cm from the pylorus along the greater curvature
- Depending on surgeon preference, stapled gastrectomy is performed with a Bougie or esophagogastrostomy scope in place

- A Bougie is a thin flexible tube inserted through the patient's esophagus, ensures adequate size of the new stomach
- Bougie size is typically larger in a duodenal switch procedure (60 Fr) when compared to a regular gastric sleeve (32–40 Fr) to limit malnutrition
- Avoid narrowing the sleeve, particularly around the incisura angularis

Duodenal Transection
- The pylorus, common bile duct, and gastroduodenal artery are identified in preparation of duodenal transection
- The duodenum is dissected approximately 2–4 cm distal to the pylorus for preservation of the pyloric valve
- After appropriate dissection, the duodenum is transected using a stapler device, and the duodenal stump is oversewn

Small Bowel Transection
- Small bowel is ran and marked approximately 75–100 cm from the ileocecal valve. This marks the location for insertion of the biliopancreatic limb
- The small bowel is then ran an additional 150–175 cm for a total of 250 cm proximal to the ileocecal valve
- The small bowel and mesentery are transected with a linear stapler at this location

Biliopancreatic Ileoileal Anastomosis
- The biliopancreatic ileoileal anastomosis is performed at the site marked 100 cm from the ileocecal valve (Y), with an end-to-side stapled anastomosis
- Modern versions of the duodenal switch leave a longer common channel than the traditional 100 cm, usually 200–300 cm of small intestine remains between the enteroenterostomy and the terminal ileum
- This connects the biliopancreatic limb to the alimentary limb to form a common channel

Duodenoileal Anastomosis
- The duodenoileal anastomosis is performed in an end-to-side fashion
- This occurs as the distal ileum or alimentary limb (Z) is divided and connected to the postpyloric duodenum
- This can be done with an absorbable or barbed suture, depending on operative approach.
- The Petersen defect, or the space between the mesentery of the alimentary limb and the transverse colon, is closed to prevent future internal hernia (Fig. 5.9)

5 Bariatric Technique and Outcomes

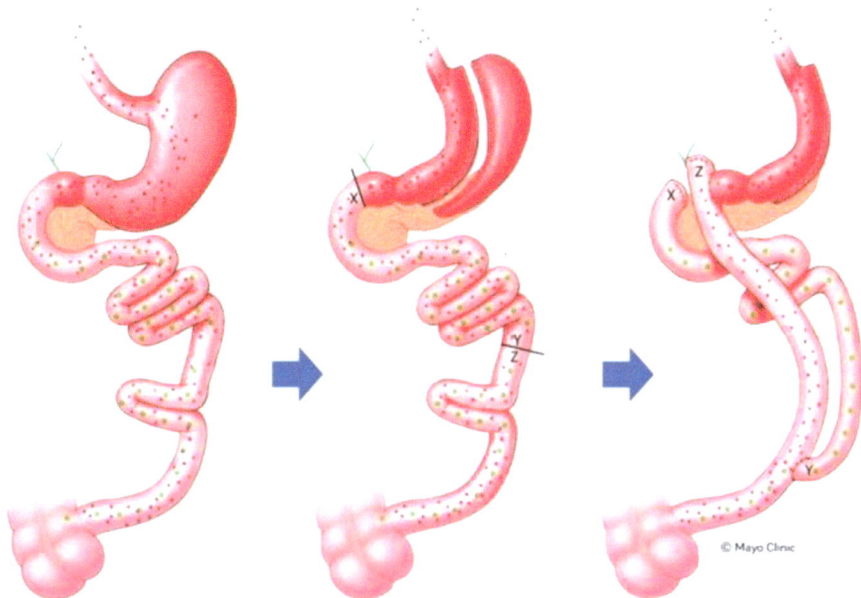

Fig. 5.9 Biliopancreatic limb (XY) and duodenal switch (Z) creation

Complications

Early

Anastomotic Leak
- Risk factors: older age, steroid use, and longer operative time
- Estimated in <1% of procedures and associated with sepsis, ICU admission, and increased morality [29]

Surgical Site Infection
- More common in open operations (7.1%) when compared to laparoscopic and robotic procedures (approximately 2%) [27]

Long-Term

Malnutrition and vitamin deficiency due to decreased dietary intake, decreased gastric acid production, and impaired absorption

- Fat-soluble vitamins (A, D, E, K)
- Vitamin B1, B9, and B12
- Zinc
- Fat malabsorption

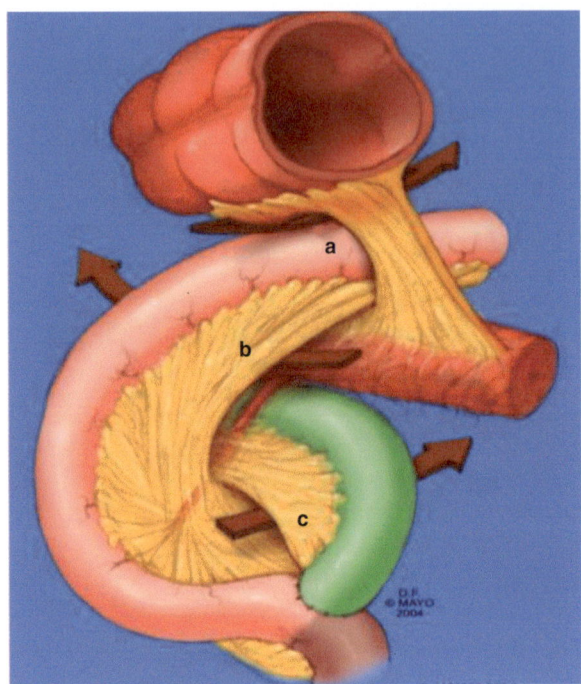

Fig. 5.10 Defects created by retrocolic approach in bypass procedures: (**a**) mesocolic, (**b**) Petersen, and (**c**) mesenteric

Internal hernia, or the passage of bowel into a mesenteric defect

- Occurs in approximately 3% of duodenal switch procedures [30]
- Higher incidence in retrocolic versus antecolic approaches due to the creation of a mesocolic defect in addition to mesenteric-mesocolic [Petersen] and jejunojejunostomy defects
- Maintain a high index of suspicion in any bypass patient presenting with symptoms of an obstruction

Mortality rates are considered similar to other bariatric procedures when evaluating high volume centers [31] (Fig. 5.10).

Outcomes

- Considered to have the greatest long-term weight loss among bariatric procedures [32]
- Improvement in comorbidities, including type 2 diabetes, hyperlipidemia, and hypertension
    - Comparable to Roux-en-Y [33]
- Higher incidence of early and long-term complications than other procedures [32]
- Estimated excess weight loss (EWL) of approximately 80% at 1 year and 72% at 10 years [24]

References

1. Seeras K. StatPearls [Internet]. 7th ed. Treasure Island: StatPearls Publishing; 2023.
2. Estimate of bariatric surgery numbers, 2011–2022. 2024. https://asmbs.org/resources/estimate-of-bariatric-surgery-numbers/. Accessed 7 Nov 2024.
3. Ponce J, DeMaria EJ, Nguyen NT, Hutter M, Sudan R, Morton JM. American Society for Metabolic and Bariatric Surgery estimation of bariatric surgery procedures in 2015 and surgeon workforce in the United States. Surg Obes Relat Dis. 2016;12:1637–9.
4. Richards W. Sabiston textbook of surgery. 21st ed. St. Louis: Elsevier; 2022.
5. Guidelines for clinical application of laparoscopic bariatric surgery – a sages publication. 2021. https://www.sages.org/publications/guidelines/guidelines-for-clinical-application-of-laparoscopic-bariatric-surgery/. Accessed 7 Nov 2024.
6. Nguyen NT, Hohmann S, Nguyen X-M, Elliott C, Masoomi H. Outcome of laparoscopic adjustable gastric banding and prevalence of band revision and explanation at academic centers: 2007–2009. Surg Obes Relat Dis. 2012;8:724–7.
7. Nasri B-N, Trainor L, Jones DB. Laparoscopic adjustable gastric band remains a safe, effective, and durable option for surgical weight loss. Surg Endosc. 2022;36:7781–8.
8. Carelli AM, Youn HA, Kurian MS, Ren CJ, Fielding GA. Safety of the laparoscopic adjustable gastric band: 7-year data from a U.S. center of excellence. Surg Endosc. 2010;24:1819–23.
9. Marceau P, et al. Biliopancreatic diversion with a new type of gastrectomy. Obes Surg. 1993;3(1):29–35.
10. Ponce J, et al. American Society for Metabolic and Bariatric Surgery estimation of bariatric surgery procedures in 2015 and surgeon workforce in the United States. Surg Obes Relat Dis. 2016;12(9):1637–9.
11. Felsenreich DM, et al. Reflux, sleeve dilation, and Barrett's esophagus after laparoscopic sleeve gastrectomy: long-term follow-up. Obes Surg. 2017;27(12):3092–101.
12. Frezza EE, et al. Complications after sleeve gastrectomy for morbid obesity. Obes Surg. 2008;19(6):684–7.
13. Peterli R, et al. Effect of laparoscopic sleeve gastrectomy vs laparoscopic Roux-en-Y gastric bypass on weight loss in patients with morbid obesity. JAMA. 2018;319(3):255.
14. Buchwald H. The evolution of metabolic/bariatric surgery. Obes Surg. 2014;24(8):1126–35. https://doi.org/10.1007/s11695-014-1354-3.
15. Townsend CM, Beauchamp RD, Evers BM, Mattox KL. Sabiston textbook of surgery: the biological basis of modern surgical practice. St. Louis: Elsevier Health Sciences; 2016.
16. Buchwald H, Avidor Y, Braunwald E, Jensen MD, Pories W, Fahrbach K, Schoelles K. Bariatric surgery: a systematic review and meta-analysis. JAMA. 2004;292(14):1724–37. https://doi.org/10.1001/jama.292.14.1724.
17. Adams TD, Davidson LE, Litwin SE, Kolotkin RL, LaMonte MJ, Pendleton RC, et al. Health benefits of gastric bypass surgery after 6 years. JAMA. 2012;308(11):1122–31. https://doi.org/10.1001/2012.jama.11164.
18. Courcoulas AP, Christian NJ, Belle SH, Berk PD, Flum DR, Garcia L, et al. Weight change and health outcomes at 3 years after bariatric surgery among individuals with severe obesity. JAMA. 2013;310(22):2416–25. https://doi.org/10.1001/jama.2013.280928.
19. Carlin AM, Zeni TM, English WJ, Hawasli AA, Genaw JA, Krause KR, et al. The comparative effectiveness of sleeve gastrectomy, gastric bypass, and adjustable gastric banding procedures for the treatment of morbid obesity. Ann Surg. 2013;257(5):791–7. https://doi.org/10.1097/SLA.0b013e3182879ded.
20. Scopinaro N, Gianetta E, Civalleri D, Bonalumi U, Bachi V. Biliopancreatic by-pass for obesity. II. Initial experience in man. Br J Surg. 1979;66(9):618–20.
21. DeMeester T, Fuchs K, Ball C, Albertucci M, Smyrk T, Marcus J. Experimental and clinical results with proximal end-to-end duodenojejunostomy for pathologic duodenogastric reflux. Ann Surg. 1987;206(4):414–26.

22. Hess DS, Hess DW. Biliopancreatic diversion with a duodenal switch. Obes Surg. 1998;8:267–82.
23. Topart P, Becouarn G. One-stage conversion of Roux-en-Y gastric bypass to a modified biliopancreatic diversion with duodenal switch using a hybrid sleeve concept. Surg Obes Relat Dis. 2016 Nov;12(9):1671–8.
24. Finno P, Osorio J, García-Ruiz-de-Gordejuela A, Casajoana A, Sorribas M, Admella V, Serrano M, Marchesini JB, Ramos AC, Pujol-Gebellí J. Single versus double-anastomosis duodenal switch: single-site comparative cohort study in 440 consecutive patients. Obes Surg. 2020;30(9):3309–16.
25. Anderson B, Gill R, de Gara C, Karmali S, Gagner M. Biliopancreatic diversion: the effectiveness of duodenal switch and its limitations. Gastroenterol Res Pract. 2013;2013(11):974762.
26. Nakanishi H, Abi Mosleh K, Al-Kordi M, Marrero K, Kermansaravi M, Davis SS Jr, Clapp B, Ghanem OM. Evaluation of long-term nutrition outcomes after duodenal switch: a systematic review and meta-analysis. Am Surg. 2024;90(3):399–410.
27. Al-Mazrou AM, Bellorin O, Dhar V, Dakin G, Afaneh C. Minimally invasive versus open duodenal switch: a nationwide retrospective analysis. Surg Endosc. 2022;36(9):7000–7.
28. Al-Mazrou AM, Cruz MV, Dakin G, Bellorin-Marin OE, Pomp A, Afaneh C. Robotic duodenal switch is associated with outcomes comparable to those of laparoscopic approach. Obes Surg. 2021;31(5):2019–29.
29. Abi Mosleh K, Corbett J, Salameh Y, Jawhar N, Puvvadi S, Davis SS Jr, Clapp B, Ghanem OM. Evaluating the incidence, risk factors and postoperative complications associated with leaks following duodenal switch procedures: an analysis of the MBSAQIP. Surg Obes Relat Dis. 2024 Sep;20(9):804–12.
30. Comeau E, Gagner M, Inabnet WB, Herron DM, Quinn TM, Pomp A. Symptomatic internal hernias after laparoscopic bariatric surgery. Surg Endosc. 2005;19(1):34–9.
31. Biertho L, Lebel S, Marceau S, Hould FS, Lescelleur O, Moustarah F, Simard S, Biron S, Marceau P. Perioperative complications in a consecutive series of 1000 duodenal switches. Surg Obes Relat Dis. 2013;9(1):63–8.
32. Maroun J, Li M, Oyefule O, Badaoui JE, McKenzie T, Kendrick M, Kellogg T, Ghanem OM. Ten year comparative analysis of sleeve gastrectomy, Roux-en-Y gastric bypass, and biliopancreatic diversion with duodenal switch in patients with BMI ≥ 50 kg/m^2. Surg Endosc. 2022;36(7):4946–55.
33. Dorman RB, Rasmus NF, al-Haddad BJ, Serrot FJ, Slusarek BM, Sampson BK, Buchwald H, Leslie DB, Ikramuddin S. Benefits and complications of the duodenal switch/biliopancreatic diversion. Surgery. 2012;152(4):758–65.

Chapter 6
Post-operative Complications Following Bariatric Surgery

Lena Egbert, James A. Madura II, Aaron Munoz, Natasha A. Sioda, and Fernando Elli

Nutritional Complications

Lena Egbert and James A. Madura II

Mechanisms Leading to Nutritional Deficiencies
- Reduced Food Intake
- Post-operatively, patients experience a reduced stomach capacity
- This physical limitation on food intake can make it challenging to consume sufficient amounts of essential nutrients
- Changes in dietary habits, namely, inadequate intake of diverse foods, also further exacerbates the risk of deficiencies
- Altered Digestion
  - Physiologic changes affect digestion and absorption post-operatively
  - Reduced stomach acid impairs release of certain nutrients from food
  - In RYGB and BPD-DS, there is delayed mixing of food with pancreatic secretions and enzymes, causing less breakdown of food into its absorbable components (See Fig. 6.1)

L. Egbert · J. A. Madura II · N. A. Sioda (✉)
Mayo Clinic, Phoenix, AZ, USA
e-mail: egbert.lena@mayo.edu; madura.james@mayo.edu; sioda.natasha@mayo.edu

A. Munoz
Mayo Clinic Alix School of Medicine, Scottsdale, AZ, USA
e-mail: munoz.aaron@mayo.edu

F. Elli
Mayo Clinic, Jacksonville, FL, USA
e-mail: elli.enrique@mayo.edu

© The Author(s), under exclusive license to Springer Nature Switzerland AG 2025
J. A. Madura II et al. (eds.), *Bariatric Surgery Clerkship*, Contemporary Surgical Clerkships, https://doi.org/10.1007/978-3-031-92964-9_6

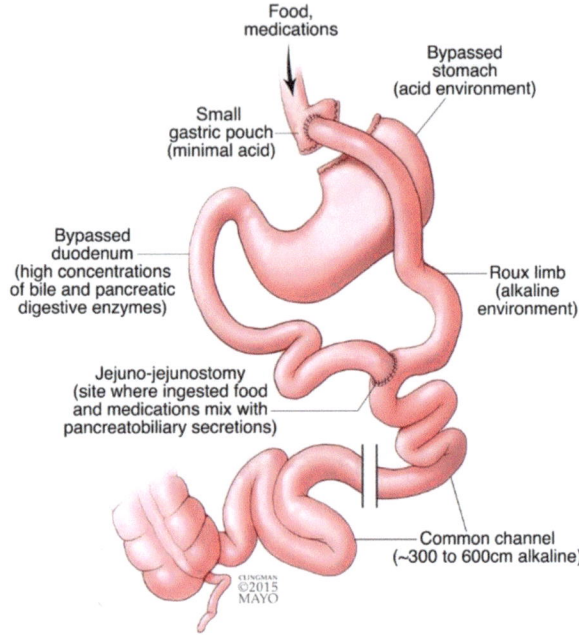

Fig. 6.1 Mechanisms leading to nutritional deficiency in Roux en Y gastric bypass

- Decreased Absorption
  - Certain procedures significantly alter the anatomy of the gastrointestinal tract, leading to malabsorption
  - In RYGB and BPD-DS, bypass of a large segment of small intestine creates a shorter common channel in which food can be absorbed (See Fig. 6.2)
- The most common deficiencies following all bariatric procedures: iron and B12

Iron

- Absorption
  - Exposure to gastric acid and pancreatic enzymes facilitates release of iron from food
  - Predominantly absorbed in the duodenum and proximal jejunum in its ionic form
- Mechanism of Deficiency
  - Reduced intake of iron-rich foods
  - Decreased exposure to gastric acid
  - Due to reconfigured anatomy in RYGB and BPD-DS, there is delayed exposure of food to pancreatic enzymes and the areas of highest iron absorption are bypassed

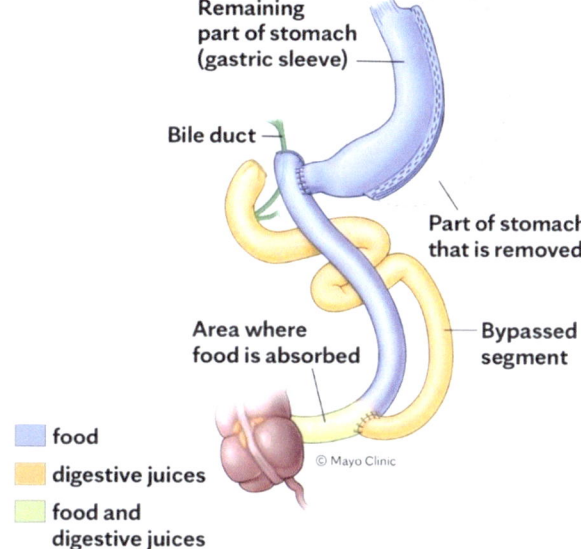

Fig. 6.2 Short common channel in biliopancreatic diversion with duodenal switch

- Symptoms of Deficiency
    - Characterized by a microcytic anemia, glossitis, koilonychia
    - Prevention: PO iron supplementation, often in a multivitamin [1–3]

Vitamin B12

- Absorption
    - Vitamin B12 is released from food by gastric acid
    - B12 binds with intrinsic factor, which is a protein produced by parietal cells in the body of the stomach
    - Vitamin B12 must complex with intrinsic factor to be absorbed in the terminal ileum
- Mechanism of Deficiency
    - In all bariatric procedures, patients may have decreased tolerance of B12-rich foods (meat, fish, dairy, eggs) due to restricted anatomy
    - Due to exclusion of a portion of the stomach in gastric sleeve, RYGB and BPD-DS, consumed food has less exposure to stomach acid and intrinsic factor
    - Due to the small bowel bypass in these RYGB and BPD-DS, there is delayed and decreased mixing of B12 with intrinsic factor

- Symptoms of Deficiency
    - Characterized by neurologic symptoms: paresthesias, subacute combined degeneration, poor cognition, depression
    - Can also cause a macrocytic anemia
    - Prevention: PO or IM Vitamin B12 supplementation [1–3]

Calcium

- Absorption
    - Vitamin D in the form of calcitriol increases transport of calcium from the bowel lumen into intestinal cells through Vitamin D-dependent calcium-binding proteins
    - The highest concentration of these calcium-binding proteins is in the duodenum and proximal jejunum
- Mechanism of Deficiency
    - Decreased levels of Vitamin D (see section "Vitamin D and other fat-soluble vitamins")
    - Malabsorption due to bypass of areas of highest absorption, the duodenum and proximal jejunum, in RYGB and BPD-DS
- Symptoms of Deficiency
    - Deficiency leads to a secondary hyperparathyroidism, releasing calcium from bones
    - This causes osteopenia which can progress to osteoporosis
    - Prevention: PO calcium carbonate or calcium citrate [1–3]

Vitamin D and Other Fat-Soluble Vitamins

- Absorption
    - Vitamin D and the other fat-soluble vitamins A, E, and K, are absorbed in the distal small intestine
    - They must form micelles with bile acids in order to be absorbed
- Mechanism of Deficiency
    - Since there is only a short common channel for food and pancreatic secretions in RYGB and BPD-DS, there is a relative deficiency of bile acids to aid in absorption of these vitamins

- Symptoms of Deficiency
    - Vitamin D: hypocalcemia and consequent osteopenia or osteoporosis as mentioned above (see section "Calcium")
    - Vitamin A: especially a concern in BPD-DS, causes poor night vision, pruritis, dry hair
    - Vitamin E: neuropathy, decreased proprioception, hemolytic anemia
    - Vitamin K: easy bleeding or bruising due to decreased activity of Vitamin K-dependent coagulation factors
    - Prevention: daily multivitamin [1–3]

Thiamine (Vitamin B1)

- Absorption
    - A water-soluble vitamin absorbed in the jejunum
    - There are low levels of storage in the body and therefore needs continuous exogenous intake to maintain normal levels
- Mechanism of Deficiency
    - Inadequate intake or patients with frequent vomiting
    - Bypass of long segment of high absorption, especially in BPD-DS
- Symptoms of Deficiency
    - Dry beriberi: peripheral neuropathy, gait ataxia, paresthesias
    - Wet beriberi: high output cardiac failure with peripheral edema
    - In severe cases, Wernicke's encephalopathy can develop: ophthalmoplegia, ataxia, nystagmus, short-term memory loss
    - Prevention: daily multivitamin [1–3]

Folate

- Absorption
    - A water-soluble vitamin absorbed throughout most of the jejunum
    - The body does not store this in large amounts and relies on a steady supply of exogenous intake
- Mechanism of Deficiency
    - Usually from insufficient intake due to the decreased volume of food consumed
    - Less absorption due to bypass of a segment of jejunum in RYGB and BPD-DS

- Symptoms of Deficiency
  - Characterized by a megaloblastic anemia, irritability, forgetfulness
  - Prevention: daily multivitamin [1–3]

Protein

- Absorption
  - Dietary proteins are broken down by pancreatic proteases and absorbed throughout the small intestine
- Mechanism of Deficiency
  - Reduced food intake since protein-rich foods are often more filling and difficult to consume in adequate amounts with restricted gastric anatomy
  - There is a short common channel in RYGB and BPD-DS, hence a diminished length of small intestine available for mixture of pancreatic enzymes with dietary protein
- Symptoms of Deficiency
  - Characterized by muscle wasting, hypoalbuminemia, poor wound healing, hair loss
  - Prevention: incorporation of protein shakes and powders into diet [1–3]

Biliary Tract Disease

Aaron Munoz and James A. Madura II

Introduction

Biliary tract disease, specifically cholesterol cholelithiasis, is a notable postoperative complication in patients who undergo bariatric surgery. Obesity and rapid weight loss are common risk factors among bariatric patients that predispose to gallstone formation and associated complications, even among patients with no prior history of gallstone disease [4, 5].

Cholelithiasis
- As many as 30–40% of bariatric surgery patients develop cholesterol gallstones, which is five times higher than in the general population [6, 7].

- Research studies suggest that 75% of gallstones precipitate within the first 2 years after surgery, with a significant majority forming within the first 6 months; approximately 7–15% progress to symptomatic cholelithiasis [8–11].
- Gallstone formation may interfere with biliary secretion, resulting in patients reporting symptoms such as nausea, anorexia, epigastric (biliary) colic, intolerance to fried or fatty foods, and diarrhea [12].
- In progressive gallstone disease, complete gallstone obstruction of the biliary duct system can precipitate life-threatening complications, such as acute cholecystitis, cholangitis, choledocholithiasis, and biliary pancreatitis [12].
- Cholecystectomy following bariatric surgery is the most common procedure in this patient population, occurring at a frequency of 6.2–14.7% [13–15].
- Although the exact mechanism remains unclear, the increased risk of symptomatic gallstone formation among bariatric patients can be attributed to several physiological changes induced by surgery and subsequent rapid weight loss.

Risk Factors for Gallstone Formation After Bariatric Surgery

Rapid or Excessive Weight Loss
- Bariatric surgery often results in significant and rapid weight loss, which is a well-documented risk factor for gallstone formation [4, 5].
- Extremely rapid weight reduction, defined as greater than 1.5 kg/week, or excessive weight reduction, defined as greater than 25% of pre-operative total body weight, increases the risk of altered bile composition [16, 17].
- The rapid mobilization of cholesterol from peripheral adipose tissue via hepatic lipolysis leads to supersaturation of bile with cholesterol.
- This cholesterol and bile acid imbalance promotes the formation of cholesterol monohydrate crystals in the gallbladder, which subsequently aggregate to form gallstones [4].

Gallbladder Hypomotility
- Reduced caloric intake and altered gastrointestinal physiology post-surgery can lead to decreased gallbladder motility.
- This hypomotility results in cholestasis and hyposecretion, which contributes to biliary sludge formation and gallstone nucleation.
- Although the exact mechanism remains unclear, post-operative reduction of oral food intake may reduce stimulation of I cells within the duodenal mucosa and contribute to biliary stasis.
- In normal human physiology, I cells secrete the peptide hormone cholecystokinin (CCK) in response to the presence of proteins and fatty acids entering the duodenal lumen.
- CCK then stimulates the release of digestive enzymes and bile from the pancreas and gallbladder, respectively, preventing cholestasis.

- Since bariatric surgery functions to reduce caloric intake and alter food bolus transit through the stomach and small intestine, reduced localized secretion of CCK within the duodenal mucosa may exacerbate gallbladder hypomotility and hyposecretion.
- However, the precise effect of bariatric surgery on CCK regulation remains unclear, since recent studies demonstrate a durable increase in postprandial CCK levels in patients who underwent RYGB or SG [18].
- Parasympathetic impulses and intraluminal releasing factors are speculated to play an as-of-yet unelucidated role in CCK homeostasis in this patient population [19].

Type of Surgery

- There is a body of evidence suggesting that the type of bariatric procedure performed may affect the incidence of gallstone formation and influence risk of subsequent cholecystectomy. Some prospective studies have found that the incidence of gallstones was 34% after RYGB and 28% after SG [6, 20].
- Similarly, a recent meta-analysis reported that SG resulted in a 35% lower incidence of gallstones and a 46% lower incidence of cholecystectomy compared to RYGB [21].
- These findings suggest that malabsorptive procedures like RYGB confer an increased risk of gallstone disease compared to restrictive approaches, potentially stemming from disparate effects on bile acid enterohepatic circulation [22].
- However, it is important to note that other prospective studies have found that both RYGB and SG increase risk for gallstone formation, albeit with no statistically significant difference between both groups [10, 23].

Ursodeoxycholic Acid Prophylaxis

- Ursodeoxycholic acid (UDCA, ursodiol) is a hydrophilic, non-toxic, secondary bile acid naturally produced by bacterial metabolism of primary bile acids in the colon [24].
- UDCA is FDA-approved for treating cholesterol gallstones, and several recent meta-analyses have demonstrated its utility as a prophylactic agent for the reduction of asymptomatic and symptomatic gallstone formation in post-operative bariatric patients undergoing weight reduction [16, 25].

- UDCA works by stimulating bile acid synthesis, decreasing hepatic secretion of cholesterol into bile, and increasing the solubility of cholesterol, thereby dissolving existing cholesterol deposits by 40–60% and preventing the formation of new gallstones [26].
- This has the benefit of improving gallbladder motility and reducing biliary stasis, thus reducing morbidity associated with bariatric surgery.
- A recent retrospective review found that patients who underwent laparoscopic sleeve gastrectomy (LSG) with UDCA prophylaxis—250 mg oral, twice daily for 6 months—had a significantly reduced risk of developing symptomatic gallstone disease that required intervention, either endoscopic retrograde cholangiopancreatography (ERCP) or cholecystectomy, compared to the non-UDCA LSG group (8.9% vs 15.8%, p = 0.022) [27].
- Similarly, a comprehensive meta-analysis of ten randomized controlled trials comparing bariatric patients receiving UDCA prophylaxis versus placebo found that a UDCA dose <600 mg/day was associated with a significantly reduced risk of gallstone formation compared to the control group (risk ratio 0.35; 95% CI 0.24–0.53; $P < 0.001$); whereas, risk reduction was not significant for a UDCA dose >600 mg/day (risk ratio 0.30; 95% CI 0.09–1.01, $P = 0.05$) [28].
- Adverse symptoms of high-dose UDCA, such as diarrhea and nausea, provide a rationale for recommending UDCA single or twice-daily doses of <600 mg/day to mitigate patient noncompliance during the recommended 6 month medication regimen [28, 29].
- UDCA (ursodiol) prophylaxis reduces the risk of gallstone formation and associated complications in bariatric patients, the 2019 update of the American Clinical Practice Guidelines For The Perioperative Nutrition, Metabolic, and Nonsurgical Support of Patients Undergoing Bariatric Procedures endorses a Grade A recommendation for oral administration of UDCA for 6 months for patients who undergo SG, RYGB, or biliopancreatic diversion without/with duodenal switch (BPD/DS): 500 mg once daily for SG and 300 mg twice a day for RYGB or BPD/DS [30].
- Despite this recommendation by the American Society for Metabolic and Bariatric Surgery, only 10.3% of bariatric surgery patients received UCDA post-operative prescriptions in 2020 [31].
- Possible explanations for UDCA under-prescription include lack of insurance coverage, financial constraints, patient reluctance, potential side effects, and high pill burden, among other reasons.
- It is crucial for providers to counsel bariatric patients about the benefits and potential side effects of UCDA prophylaxis, as well as strategies to mitigate medication noncompliance.
- It is equally important that providers work with insurance companies to expand coverage and accessibility of UCDA for patients of all income demographics.

Early and Late Dumping Syndrome

Natasha A. Sioda and James A. Madura II

Introduction

Dumping syndrome is a common complication seen in patients that have undergone esophageal, bariatric, and gastric surgery. The documented incidence of dumping syndrome is variable with a documented range of 13–16% in post-operative LRYGB patients [32–34]. Dumping syndrome has also been documented in patients that have undergone sleeve gastrectomy, but more data still needs to be gathered to determine overall incidence [35, 36].

Early Dumping Syndrome

- Tyically occurs within 1 h of eating.
- This is due to the fast passage of hyperosmolar contents into the duodenum which leads to a large influx of fluid into the intestines.
- This rapid shift results in a vasoactive response from release of gastrointestinal hormones.
- Symptoms often reported include flushing, palpitations, tachycardia, diaphoresis, hypotension, syncope, abdominal pain, nausea, and bloating [36, 37].

Late Dumping Syndrome

- Late dumping syndrome is also known as postprandial hyperinsulinemic hypoglycemia.
- It occurs between 1–3 h after eating.
- The etiology of late dumping is thought to be due to a surge in insulin release after rapid intestinal absorption of glucose which results in hypoglycemia [36, 37].

Diagnosis

Oral Glucose Challenge

- An oral glucose challenge can be used during the diagnostic workup for dumping syndrome.
- Patients fast for 10 h overnight. The patient's heart rate and blood pressure are then measured before, during, and after they consume 50 g of glucose in addition to hematocrit levels.
- A test is considered positive for early dumping syndrome if a patient's heart rate increases by at least 10 beats/min or hematocrit increases by more than 3%.
- For late dumping syndrome, blood glucose is measured and hypoglycemia measured 1–2 h after consumption is suggestive of late dumping syndrome [37, 38].

Differential Diagnosis

Gastroparesis
- In some instances, dumping syndrome can be confused for gastroparesis or irritable bowel syndrome (IBS).
- One study reported that 37% of patients with dumping syndrome were diagnosed with gastroparesis.
- Radionuclide scintigraphy can distinguish between the two diagnoses [39].

Irritable Bowel Syndrome (IBS)
- IBS can be distinguished from dumping syndrome using the Rome III diagnostic criteria.
- Using this reference patients with IBS must present with two of three following criteria for at least 3 months: changes in stool consistency, stool frequency, and relief of abdominal pain following defecation [38].

Further workup with endoscopy, colonoscopy, stool analysis, and blood work can be used to aid diagnosis.

Treatment

Behavioral Modification
- The initial treatment for early dumping syndrome is behavioral modification.
- Patients are counseled to eat small frequent meals and avoid foods with high sugar content.

- Meals consisting of proteins, fats, fiber, and complex carbohydrates are encouraged as they can slow digestion and aid in preventing symptoms.
- Laying supine for 30 min after meals has also been thought to potentially slow gastric emptying [36–38].

Pharmaceutical Agents
- Pharmaceutical agents to slow gastric emptying have also been proposed in patients that experience symptoms despite behavior modification.
- Acarbose is an alpha-glycosidase hydrolase inhibitor that slows the breakdown of carbohydrates reducing overall absorption and subsequent insulin surge. Unabsorbed carbohydrates may increase symptoms of diarrhea and flatulence and should be monitored [37, 38].
- Somatostatin analogs such as, octreotide (short-acting) and lanreotide or pasireotid(long-acting) have been used to slow gastric emptying, inhibit hormones that cause splanchnic vasodilation [36–38].
- Anticholinergics can slow gastric emptying and is an antispasmodic which can help relieve some of the abdominal pain related to dumping syndrome [38].
- In some studies, nifedipine and diazoxide have shown some success in decreasing late dumping symptoms through decreasing insulin release from the pancreas [37, 38].

Marginal Ulcers

Natasha A. Sioda and James A. Madura II

Introduction

Marginal ulcers occur at or near a gastroenterostomy anastomosis and can be present on either side of the anastomosis. The average reported prevalence of marginal ulcers following a roux-en-Y gastric bypass is 4.6–8% [37, 40].

Pathogenesis

Early Ulceration
- Thought to be related to technical factors such as ischemia and tension on the anastomosis.
- Acid likely plays a role but there should not be much parietal cell mass in a properly constructed GBP pouch.
- Constructing anastomoses with non-absorbable suture has also been shown to be associated with ulceration [41]. Late Ulcerations

- Defined as over 1 year post-operatively
- Considered likely "environmental" ulcers; meaning there is something other than the technical construction that is at play.
- In these cases, medications, smoking, alcohol ingestion, change in dietary habits and H. pylori infection should be entertained as possible culprits [41].

Distal Ulcers
- When ulcers occur to the distal aspect of the anastomosis, it is postulated that the cause is secondary to acid to the small bowel mucosa.

Proximal Ulcers
- When ulcers occurs proximally it is thought to be due to ischemia, bile reflux, stasis, foreign body.

Predisposing Factors

- The use of NSAIDs, presence of H. pylori, diabetes, corticosteroids, previous history of peptic ulcer, deep vein thrombosis, alcohol consumption, and smoking are risk factors for marginal ulcer development [40, 42].

Symptoms

- Symptom presentation is variable.
- Reported symptoms include upper abdominal discomfort, hematochezia, nausea, and vomiting.
- It is predicted that approximately 25% of patients with marginal ulcers are asymptomatic [42]

Diagnosis

- Patients presenting with symptoms concerning for a marginal ulcer should undergo assessment with an upper endoscopy for diagnosis.

Treatment and Prevention

- The first step of treatment is removal of modifiable risk factors. This can include smoking cessation, discontinuation of NSAID use, and H. pylori eradication.

- Studies have shown that proton pump inhibitors (PPIs) reduce incidence of marginal ulcers. The exact duration and dose is still debated. The majority of marginal ulcers resolve or improve with use of PPI. Approximately 11.5% of patients experience persistent symptoms and are followed up with endoscopy [42].
- Approximately 12% of patients with marginal ulcers undergo revisional surgery of the gastrojejunostomic site to resect the area containing the marginal ulcer(s) [42].

Bleeding

- In most cases a bleeding marginal ulcer can be managed either endoscopically or with angioembolization without need for surgery [37].
- In patients with persistent bleeding, surgery may be performed to control bleeding in the form of oversewing the vessel or resection of anastomotic site.

Perforation

- A severe complication related to marginal ulcers is gastrointestinal perforation.
- In unstable and high risk patients, a patch closure is the preferred surgical treatment.
- In stable patients and low risk patients, the anastomotic site may be resected [37].

Gastrointestinal Leaks and Gastro-Gastric Fistulas

Natasha A. Sioda and Fernando Elli

Gastrointestinal Leaks

Introduction

Gastrointestinal leak is one of the most severe complications following bariatric surgery. The overall rate of incidence is low with an estimated leak rate <1%. The reported leak rate following LSG ranges from 0–8% and 0.1%–8.3% after LRYGB [43]. The most common site of gastrointestinal leak after a LRYGB is at the GJ. In sleeve gastrectomy, it is often observed to the proximal third of the gastric staple line [43].

Pre-disposing Factors

- Leaks typically occur after hospital discharge 5–15 days post-operatively [44, 45].
- Patients that are older and chronically ill have a higher risk of developing a gastro-intestinal leak prior to discharge [45].
- Predisposing factors that increase risk of gastrointestinal leak are a history of oxygen dependency, hypoalbuminemia, sleep apnea, hypertension, and diabetes [43].
- Data also suggests that surgeon operative skill impacts overall leak rate with more experienced surgeons reporting a smaller leak rate [43, 46].
- Studies have demonstrated no difference in leak rate based off type of anastomosis or stapling device used [46].

Diagnosis

- Surgeons often perform an intraoperative leak test at time of bariatric surgery to detect a gastrointestinal leak.
- It consists of distension of the gastric pouch with air using either an orogastric tube or endoscope.
- The pouch is then submerged with irrigated saline.
- The presence of bubbles is indicative of a leak and the staple line is often oversewn at site of detected leak.
- The use of intra-abdominal surgical drains for gastrointestinal leak prevention has not been shown to have substantial benefit in studies [43].
- In stable patients with a suspected leak post-operatively a contrast swallow test can be performed.
- This is an x-ray study that follows oral contrast from the mouth through the small intestine.
- If there is a leak , there will be extravasation of contrast [43].
- The routine use of post-operative contrast swallow studies is not well supported with data suggesting that it does lead to earlier detection rates [43, 44].

Treatment

- Gastrointestinal leaks are repaired surgically with either revision or temporizing measures in unstable patients.
- In select patients with small gastrointestinal leaks, conservative management with antibiotics, bowel rest, parenterial nutrition may be an option.
- In hospitals with advanced endoscopic capabilities, small gastrointestinal leaks may be controlled endoscopically with clips and tissue sealants, but more studies need to be conducted to demonstrate utility [47].

Gastrogastric Fistula

Introduction

Gastrogastric fistulas (GGF) are an abnormal connection between the gastric pouch and gastric remnant. Gastrogastric fistulas occur in approximately 1–6% of patients that underwent a roux-en-Y Gastric bypass [48].

Symptoms

- Patients with GGFs may be asymptomatic or present with nonspecific symptoms.
- Symptoms can include nausea, vomiting, abdominal bloating, abdominal pain, and inadequate weight gain [48].

Diagnosis

- EGD, CT scans with oral contrast, and upper GI series can all be used to identify a GGF.
- Imaging will demonstrate presence of contrast or air in the gastric remnant.
- EGD can help identify the exact location of the GGF which can assist with operative planning [48].

Etiology

- The predicted cause of gastrogastric fistulas is either a post-operative leak, suspected micro-leak, or a marginal ulcer [49].

Treatment

- The initial treatment for GGF often includes conservative management with H. pylori eradication, NSAID/smoking cessation, high dose PPI, and sucralfate.
- The goal is to reduce gastric acid secretion which may aid in spontaneous closure without need for invasive procedures.
- The predicted spontaneous resolution of GGF with conservative management is approximately 20% [50].
- The most definitive approach to GGF closure includes surgical repair, but endoscopic management has been adopted.
- Endoscopic procedures include use of fibrin sealant, endoclips, and endoscopic suturing [48, 50, 51].

- The longterm durability of endoscopic intervention is limited and is typically reserved for smaller caliber fistulous tracts <1 cm in diameter [51].
- Surgical management of GGF involves excision of the fistula with or without preservation of the gastrojejunal anastomosis depending on the location and etiology of the GGF [48].

Internal Hernias

Natasha A. Sioda and Fernando Elli

- Internal hernia is defined as protrusion of intra-abdominal organs through a peritoneal or mesenteric defect.
- The incidence of internal hernia following LRYGB is approximately 1–6% [52].
- Delay in diagnosis of an internal hernia can lead to higher morbidity and mortality [52].
- The incidence of internal hernia is higher in patient's with a retrocolic LRYGB compared to an antecolic LRYGB.
- With the antecolic approach, there are two particular defects at risk for internal herniation.
- The first defect is posterior to the roux limb commonly referred to as Petersen defect and the second defect is the mesentery defect resulting from the jejunojejunostomy creation [53].

Prevention

- There is debate regarding the efficacy of closing the mesenteric and Petersen's defect during initial operation to prevent future internal hernias.
- There have been some studies that demonstrate reduction in internal hernia occurrence with closure of defects [53, 54].
- We would recommend considering closure of mesenteric and Petersen's defect at time of initial operation

Symptoms

- Symptoms of an internal hernias are variable ranging from patients being entirely asymptomatic to having nonspecific abdominal pain to significant obstructive and peritoneal signs.

- More severe cases of internal hernia can present with incarceration and strangulation of intra-abdominal contents.
- The incidence of internal hernia most often occurs within 1–2 years following surgery which aligns with time period with the most significant weight loss [53].

Diagnosis

- CT findings of an internal hernia often demonstrate mesenteric swirling and loops of bowel in the left upper quadrant [55].
- A meta-analysis demonstrated that CT scan has a pooled sensitivity of 82% and specificity of 84.8% in diagnosing an internal hernia [56].
- Within this meta-analysis, mesenteric swirl sign, venous congestion and mesenteric edema had the highest sensitivity for diagnosing an internal hernia [56].

Treatment

- Variable and nonspecific presentation of an internal hernia may lead to a delay in treatment.
- If not treated, internal hernia complicated by strangulation has an overall mortality over 50% [55].
- Treatment is surgical exploration in order to reduce hernia contents and may necessitate bowel resection depending on the viability of the herniated bowel contents.

Venous Thromboembolism

Natasha A. Sioda and Fernando Elli

- Venous thromboembolism is the leading cause of death following bariatric surgery [57].
- Deep venous thrombosis (DVT) occur in 1–3% of patients after bariatric surgery [57].
- Pulmonary embolism (PE) occurs in approximately 0.1–2% of patients after bariatric surgery [57].
- Most events of VTE occur post-operatively after a patient has been discharged from the hospital.
- With approximately 73–84% of episodes of VTE occurring after hospitalization [57].

Risk Factors

- Smoking, greater age, increased BMI, male sex have been shown to be post-operative risk factors for VTE in bariatric patients [58].
- Surgery related factors that increase post-operative risk for VTE include longer operative time, post-operative anastomotic leak, and open procedures [58].

VTE Prophylaxis

- Patients who undergo bariatric surgery are at moderate to high risk for venous thromboembolism (VTE).
- Because of their risk, they should undergo both mechanical prophylaxis with SCDs, early ambulation, and chemoprophylaxis after surgery [46].
- The Michigan Bariatric Surgery Collaborative demonstrated that patients who received low molecular weight heparin had lower rates of VTE as compared to patients who received unfractioned heparin [59].
- VTE prophylaxis practice is variable and there is currently no consensus on the dosage, frequency, and duration that patients should receive post-operatively [57].

References

1. Alvarez-Leite JI. Nutrient deficiencies secondary to bariatric surgery. Curr Opin Clin Nutr Metab Care. 2004;7(5):569–75.
2. Bal BS, Finelli FC, Shope TR, Koch TR. Nutritional deficiencies after bariatric surgery. Nat Rev Endocrinol. 2012;8(9):544–56. https://doi.org/10.1038/nrendo.2012.48.
3. Parrott J, Frank L, Rabena R, Craggs-Dino L, Isom KA, Greiman L. American Society for Metabolic and Bariatric Surgery integrated health nutritional guidelines for the surgical weight loss patient 2016 update: micronutrients. Surg Obes Relat Dis. 2017;13(5):727–41. https://doi.org/10.1016/j.soard.2016.12.018.
4. Albaugh VL, Banan B, Ajouz H, Abumrad NN, Flynn CR. Bile acids and bariatric surgery. Mol Asp Med. 2017;56:75–89.
5. Gustafsson U, Benthin L, Granström L, Groen AK, Sahlin S, Einarsson C. Changes in gallbladder bile composition and crystal detection time in morbidly obese subjects after bariatric surgery. Hepatology. 2005;41(6):1322–8.
6. Yuan S, Gill D, Giovannucci EL, Larsson SC. Obesity, type 2 diabetes, lifestyle factors, and risk of gallstone disease: a Mendelian randomization investigation. Clin Gastroenterol Hepatol. 2022;20(3):e529–e37.
7. Adams LB, Chang C, Pope J, Kim Y, Liu P, Yates A. Randomized, prospective comparison of ursodeoxycholic acid for the prevention of gallstones after sleeve gastrectomy. Obes Surg. 2016;26(5):990–4.
8. Nabil TM, Khalil AH, Gamal K. Effect of oral ursodeoxycholic acid on cholelithiasis following laparoscopic sleeve gastrectomy for morbid obesity. Surg Obes Relat Dis. 2019;15(6):827–31.
9. Altieri MS, Yang J, Nie L, Docimo S, Talamini M, Pryor AD. Incidence of cholecystectomy after bariatric surgery. Surg Obes Relat Dis. 2018;14(7):992–6.

10. Andrés-Imaz A, Martí-Gelonch L, Eizaguirre-Letamendia E, Asensio-Gallego JI, Enríquez-Navascués JM. Incidence and risk factors for de novo cholelithiasis after bariatric surgery. Cir Esp (Engl Ed). 2021;99(9):648–54.
11. Coupaye M, Calabrese D, Sami O, Msika S, Ledoux S. Evaluation of incidence of cholelithiasis after bariatric surgery in subjects treated or not treated with ursodeoxycholic acid. Surg Obes Relat Dis. 2017;13(4):681–5.
12. Portenier DD, Grant JP, Blackwood HS, Pryor A, McMahon RL, DeMaria E. Expectant management of the asymptomatic gallbladder at Roux-en-Y gastric bypass. Surg Obes Relat Dis. 2007;3(4):476–9.
13. Portincasa P, Moschetta A, Petruzzelli M, Palasciano G, Di Ciaula A, Pezzolla A. Symptoms and diagnosis of gallbladder stones. Best Pract Res Clin Gastroenterol. 2006;20(6):1017–29.
14. Magouliotis DE, Christodoulidis G, Zacharoulis D. The necessity for routine administration of ursodeoxycholic acid after bariatric surgery. Obes Surg. 2020;30(6):2421–2.
15. Magouliotis DE, Tasiopoulou VS, Svokos AA, Svokos KA, Chatedaki C, Sioka E, et al. Ursodeoxycholic acid in the prevention of gallstone formation after bariatric surgery: an updated systematic review and meta-analysis. Obes Surg. 2017;27(11):3021–30.
16. Wrzesinski A, CorrÊA JM, Fernandes TMB, Monteiro LF, Trevisol FS, do Nascimento RR. Complications requiring hospital management after bariatric surgery. Arq Bras Cir Dig (São Paulo). 2015;28:3–6.
17. Liddle RA, Goldstein RB, Saxton J. Gallstone formation during weight-reduction dieting. Arch Intern Med. 1989;149(8):1750–3.
18. Weinsier RL, Wilson LJ, Lee J. Medically safe rate of weight loss for the treatment of obesity: a guideline based on risk of gallstone formation. Am J Med. 1995;98(2):115–7.
19. Peterli R, Steinert RE, Woelnerhanssen B, Peters T, Christoffel-Courtin C, Gass M, et al. Metabolic and hormonal changes after laparoscopic Roux-en-Y gastric bypass and sleeve gastrectomy: a randomized, prospective trial. Obes Surg. 2012;22(5):740–8.
20. Steinert RE, Feinle-Bisset C, Asarian L, Horowitz M, Beglinger C, Geary N. Ghrelin, CCK, GLP-1, and PYY(3-36): secretory controls and physiological roles in eating and glycemia in health, obesity, and after RYGB. Physiol Rev. 2017;97(1):411–63.
21. Sugerman HJ, Brewer WH, Shiffman ML, Brolin RE, Fobi MAL, Linner JH, et al. A multicenter, placebo-controlled, randomized, double-blind, prospective trial of prophylactic ursodiol for the prevention of gallstone formation following gastric-bypass-induced rapid weight loss. Am J Surg. 1995;169(1):91–7.
22. Wan Q, Zhao R, Chen Y, Wang Y, Wu Y, Wu X. Comparison of the incidence of cholelithiasis after sleeve gastrectomy and Roux-en-Y gastric bypass: a meta-analysis. Surg Obes Relat Dis. 2021;17(6):1198–205.
23. Abdallah E, Emile SH, Elfeki H, Fikry M, Abdelshafy M, Elshobaky A, et al. Role of ursodeoxycholic acid in the prevention of gallstone formation after laparoscopic sleeve gastrectomy. Surg Today. 2017;47(7):844–50.
24. Fearon NM, Kearns EC, Kennedy CA, Conneely JB, Heneghan HM. The impact of ursodeoxycholic acid on gallstone disease after bariatric surgery: a meta-analysis of randomized control trials. Surg Obes Relat Dis. 2022;18(1):77–84.
25. Chiang JY. Bile acid metabolism and signaling. Compr Physiol. 2013;3(3):1191–212.
26. Ward JBJ, Lajczak NK, Kelly OB, O'Dwyer AM, Giddam AK, Ní Gabhann J, et al. Ursodeoxycholic acid and lithocholic acid exert anti-inflammatory actions in the colon. Am J Physiol Gastrointest Liver Physiol. 2017;312(6):G550–8.
27. Mulliri A, Menahem B, Alves A, Dupont B. Ursodeoxycholic acid for the prevention of gallstones and subsequent cholecystectomy after bariatric surgery: a meta-analysis of randomized controlled trials. J Gastroenterol. 2022;57(8):529–39.
28. Stellaard F, Lütjohann D. Dynamics of the enterohepatic circulation of bile acids in healthy humans. Am J Physio Gastrointest Liver Physiol. 2021;321(1):G55–66.

29. Hossain I, Brodie J, O'Brien E, Tedman-Aucoin K, Lawlor D, Murphy R, et al. Ursodeoxycholic acid for prevention of gallstone disease after laparoscopic sleeve gastrectomy: an Atlantic Canada perspective. Surg Endosc. 2023;37(7):5236–40.
30. Mechanick JI, Apovian C, Brethauer S, Garvey WT, Joffe AM, Kim J, et al. Clinical practice guidelines for the perioperative nutrition, metabolic, and nonsurgical support of patients undergoing bariatric procedures—2019. Update. 2019;25:1–75.
31. Coogan AC, Williams MD, Krishnan V, Skertich NJ, Becerra AZ, Sarran M, et al. Ursodiol prescriptions following bariatric surgery: National prescribing trends and outcomes. Obes Surg. 2023;33(8):2361–7.
32. Nielsen JB, Pedersen AM, Gribsholt SB, Svensson E, Richelsen B. Prevalence, severity, and predictors of symptoms of dumping and hypoglycemia after Roux-en-Y gastric bypass. Surg Obes Relat Dis. 2016;12(8):1562–8.
33. Laurenius A, Olbers T, Naslund I. Dumping syndrome following gastric bypass: validation of the dumping syndrome rating scale. Obes Surg. 2013;17(11):740–55.
34. Mallory GN, Macrgregor AM, Rand C. The influence of dumping on weight loss after gastric restrictive surgery for morbid obesity. Obes Surg. 1996;6(6):474–8.
35. Ahmad A, Kornrich DB, Krasner H, Eckardt S, Ahmad Z, Braslow A, Broggelwirth B. Prevalence of dumping syndrome after laparoscopic sleeve gastrectomy and comparison with laparoscopic Roux-en-Y gastric bypass. Obes Surg. 2019;29(5):1506–13.
36. Tack J, Deloose E. Complications of bariatric surgery: dumping syndrome, reflux and vitamin deficiencies. Best Pract Res Clin Gastroenterol. 2014;28(4):741–9.
37. Cameron JL, Cameron AM. Current surgical therapy. 13th ed. Available from: Elsevier eBooks+. Philadelphia: Elsevier – OHCE; 2019
38. Berg P, McCallum R. Dumping syndrome: a review of the current concepts of pathophysiology, diagnosis, and treatment. Dig Dis Sci. 2016;61(1):11–8.
39. Berg P, et al. Dumping syndrome, updated perspectives on etiologies and diagnosis. Pract Gastroenterol. 2014;38:30–8.
40. Salame M, Jawhar N, Belluzzi A, Al-Kordi M, Storm AC, Abu Dayyeh BK, Ghanem OM. Marginal ulcers after Roux-en-Y gastric bypass: etiology, diagnosis, and management. J Clin Med. 2023;12(13):4336. https://doi.org/10.3390/jcm12134336. PMID: 37445371; PMCID: PMC10342478.
41. Sacks B, Mattar S, Qureshi F, Eid G, Collins J, Barinas-Mitchell E, Schauer P, Ramanathan R. Incidence of marginal ulcers and the use of absorbable anastomotic sutures in laparoscopic Roux-en-Y gastric bypass. Surg Obes Relat Dis. 2006;2(1):11–8.
42. Süsstrunk J, Wartmann L, Mattiello D, Köstler T, Zingg U. Incidence and prognostic factors for the development of symptomatic and asymptomatic marginal ulcers after Roux-en-Y gastric bypass procedures. Obes Surg. 2021;31:3005–14.
43. Alizadeh RF, Li S, Inaba C, Penalosa P, Hinojosa MW, Smith BR, Stamos MJ, Nguyen NT. Risk factors for gastrointestinal leak after bariatric surgery: MBASQIP analysis. J Am Coll Surg. 2018;227(1):135–41.
44. Trac J, Balas M, Gee D, Hutter MM, Jung JJ. Does routine upper gastrointestinal swallow study after metabolic and bariatric surgery lead to earlier diagnosis of leak? Surg Obes Relat Dis. 2024;20(8):767–73.
45. Spaniolas K, Kasten KR, Sippey ME, Pender JR, Chapman WH, Pories WJ. Pulmonary embolism and gastrointestinal leak following bariatric surgery: when do major complications occur? Surg Obes Relat Dis. 2016;12(2):379–83.
46. Townsend CM. Sabiston textbook of surgery. 21st ed. Available from: Elsevier eBooks+. Philadelphia: Elsevier – OHCE; 2021
47. Rogalski P, Daniluk J, Baniukiewicz A, Wroblewski E, Dabrowski A. Endoscopic management of gastrointestinal perforations, leaks and fistulas. World J Gastroenterol. 2015;21(37):10542–52.
48. Chahine E, Kassir R, Dirani M, et al. Surgical management of gastrogastric fistula after Roux-en-Y gastric bypass: 10-year experience. Obes Surg. 2018;28:939–44.

49. Pauli E, Beshir H, Mathew A. Gastrogastric fistulae following gastric bypass surgery—clinical recognition and treatment. Curr Gastroenterol Rep. 2014;16:405.
50. Gumbs AA, Duffy AJ, Bell RL. Management of gastrogastric fistula after laparoscopic Roux-en-Y gastric bypass. Surg Obes Relat Dis. 2006;2(2):117–21.
51. Fernandez-Esparrach G, Lautz DB, Thompson CC. Endoscopic repair of gastrogastric fistula after Roux-en-Y gastric bypass: a less-invasive approach. Surg Obes Relat Dis. 2010;6(3):282–8.
52. Nimeri AA, Maasher A, Al Shaban T, Salim E, Gamaleldin MM. Internal hernia following laparoscopic Roux-en-Y gastric bypass: prevention and tips for intra-operative management. Obes Surg. 2016;26(9):2255–6.
53. Blockhuys M, Gypen B, Heyman S, Valk J, van Sprundel F, Hendrickx L. Internal hernia after laparoscopic gastric bypass: effect of closure of the Petersen defect – single-center study. Obes Surg. 2019;1:70–5.
54. Stenberg E, Ottosson J, Magnuson A, et al. Long-term safety and efficacy of closure of mesenteric defects in laparoscopic gastric bypass surgery: a randomized clinical trial. JAMA Surg. 2023;158(7):709–17.
55. Martin LC, Merkle EM, Thompson WM. Review of internal hernias: radiographic and clinical findings. AJR Am J Roentgenol. 2006;186(3):703–17.
56. Nawas MA, Oor JE, Goense L, Hosman SFM, van der Hoeven EJRJ, Wijffels NAT, Riele WWT, Takkenberg M, Wiezer MJ, Derksen WJM. The diagnostic accuracy of abdominal computed tomography in diagnosing internal herniation following Roux-en-Y gastric bypass surgery: a systematic review and meta-analysis. Ann Surg. 2022;275(5):856–63.
57. Giannopoulos S, Kalantar Motamedi SM, Athanasiadis DI, Clapp B, Lyo V, Ghanem O, Edwards M, Puzziferri N, Stefanidis D. ASMBS Research Committee. Venous thromboembolism (VTE) prophylaxis after bariatric surgery: a national survey of MBSAQIP director practices. Surg Obes Relat Dis. 2023;19(8):799–807.
58. Bartlett MA, Mauck KF, Daniels PR. Prevention of venous thromboembolism in patients undergoing bariatric surgery. Vasc Health Risk Manag. 2015;11:461–77.
59. Birkmeyer NJO, Finks JF, Carlin AM, et al. Comparative effectiveness of unfractionated and low-molecular-weight heparin for prevention of venous thromboembolism following bariatric surgery. Arch Surg. 2012;147(11):994–8.

Chapter 7
Alternatives to Bariatric Surgery

Isabella Reitz, Fernando Elli, Lindsey Trinchet, and Natasha A. Sioda

Weight Loss Medications

Isabella Reitz and Fernando Elli

Introduction

Weight loss medication can be an integral component of a patient's overall treatment plan for managing obesity. As of 2024, the FDA has approved nine anti-obesity drugs. According to current guidelines, weight loss medication is recommended for individuals who, despite making lifestyle changes, have a body mass index (BMI) of 30 kg/m^2 or higher, or a BMI of 27 kg/m^2 with associated obesity-related comorbidities. For optimal results, these medications should be used in conjunction with ongoing dietary adjustments and exercise [1–6].

I. Reitz · L. Trinchet
Mayo Clinic Alix School of Medicine, Scottsdale, AZ, USA
e-mail: reitz.isabella@mayo.edu; trinchet.lindsey@mayo.edu

F. Elli
Mayo Clinic, Jacksonville, FL, USA
e-mail: elli.enrique@mayo.edu

N. A. Sioda (✉)
Mayo Clinic, Phoenix, AZ, USA
e-mail: sioda.natasha@mayo.edu

© The Author(s), under exclusive license to Springer Nature Switzerland AG 2025
J. A. Madura II et al. (eds.), *Bariatric Surgery Clerkship*, Contemporary Surgical Clerkships, https://doi.org/10.1007/978-3-031-92964-9_7

GLP-1 Agonists

Glucagon-Like Peptide-1 (GLP-1)
- Incretin hormone that is secreted postprandially from the gut
- Regulates blood glucose by:
  - Inhibiting glucagon secretion.
  - Enhancing insulin secretion in a glucose-dependent manner.
- Slows gastric emptying, contributing to postprandial satiety and reduced appetite.
- Acts on the hypothalamus, limbic system, and cortex to decrease hunger and food intake

GLP-1 Receptor Agonists
- Administered via weekly subcutaneous injections.
- Effective for managing type 2 diabetes and obesity.
- Weight loss results:
  - Patients lose 10–20% of their total body weight on average.
  - Current studies suggest that GLP-1 agonists may have a more pronounced effect on weight loss in non-diabetic patients compared to those with diabetes.
- Cardiovascular benefits:
  - Reductions in major adverse cardiovascular events (MACE), including cardiovascular death, myocardial infarction, and stroke.
  - FDA-approved for secondary cardiovascular prevention in patients with type 2 diabetes.
- Associated with gastrointestinal side effects, including nausea and vomiting.
- Potential risks for more serious conditions include:
  - Pancreatitis
  - Bowel obstruction
  - Pancreatic cancer
  - Thyroid cancer
- Expensive and may pose challenges with insurance coverage.
- Access issues may delay treatment.

FDA-Approved GLP-1 Agonists
- Liraglutide:
- Approved in 2010 as Victoza for type 2 diabetes mellitus (T2DM) at doses of 1.2 or 1.8 mg.
- A higher dose formulation (3 mg) was introduced in 2014 as Saxenda for weight management.
- Expanded indication in 2020 to include adolescents aged 12 to 17 years old who weigh more than 60 kg.

- Clinical studies show significant long-term weight loss when combined with moderate-to-vigorous exercise.
- Semaglutide:
  - Approved in 2017 as Ozempic for T2DM.
  - A higher dose (2.4 mg) was approved in 2021 as Wegovy for weight loss.
  - Wegovy achieves a weight reduction of 10–20% as shown in the STEP clinical trials.
  - Designed to remain active in the body longer, leading to a sustained 12.5% weight reduction over 2 years compared to placebo.
- Tirzepatide:
  - First-in-class dual agonist targeting both GLP-1 and glucose-dependent insulinotropic peptide (GIP) receptors.
  - Approved for T2DM as Mounjaro in 2022.
  - Approved for weight loss as Zepbound (2.5 mg) in 2023.
  - Studies show more significant weight loss with Zepbound compared to other GLP-1 agonists.

Emerging GLP-1 Receptor Agonists
- Benaglutide:
- Recombinant human GLP-1 analog approved in China.
- Demonstrates efficacy in lowering HbA1c and fasting plasma glucose while reducing body weight.
- Orforglipron and Retatrutide:
  - Both show promising results in reducing body weight.
  - Currently in phase 3 clinical trials [1–6].

Other Weight Loss Medication

Phentermine
- Available under brand names Adipex-P and Lomaira.
- One of the oldest anti-obesity medications, FDA-approved in 1959.
- Indicated for short-term use up to 12 weeks for weight management in eligible individuals.
- Functions by stimulating the release of norepinephrine, which reduces appetite.
- Typically results in a weight loss of about 5% of a patient's body weight.
- Limitations:
  - Loss of lean muscle mass
  - Metabolic disturbances
  - Headaches

- Dizziness
  - Increased heart rate and palpitations
  - Insomnia
  - Exacerbation of anxiety
  - Potential for misuse due to sympathomimetic properties.
- Requires caution in patients with:
  - Coronary heart disease.
  - Hypertension.
  - Increased risk of medication misuse.

Phentermine/Topiramate
- FDA-approved in 2012.
- Available in four dosing combinations:
  - 3.75/23 mg
  - 7.5/46 mg
  - 11.25/69 mg
  - 15/92 mg
- Administered daily
- The dose is gradually escalated every 2–12 weeks as long as weight reduction exceeds 5%.
- Phentermine works as a sympathomimetic agent.
- Topiramate works as a gamma-aminobutyric acid (GABA) modulator and dopamine/norepinephrine reuptake inhibitor.
  - Mitigates some of phentermine's side effects.
  - Promotes taste aversion and reduces caloric intake.
- 52-week CONQUER randomized clinical trial showed:
  - Placebo-subtracted weight loss of 6.6% at the mid-dose.
  - Placebo-subtracted weight loss of 8.6% at the maximum dose.
- Use with caution in patients with cardiovascular conditions due to potential risks.
- Topiramate-related side effects:
  - Sedation
  - Kidney stones
  - Dry mouth
- Monitor for neuropsychiatric side effects such as:
  - Depression
  - Suicidal thoughts
  - Cognitive changes
- Associated with an increased risk of fetal cleft palate so contraindicated in pregnant women.

Orlistat

- FDA-approved in 1999 for weight management at a dose of 120 mg.
- Initially approved for use in adolescents aged 12–16.
- A lower dose formulation of 60 mg was introduced in 2007 as Alli, available over-the-counter (OTC) for overweight adult patients.
- Inhibits gastrointestinal and pancreatic lipases, therefore reducing absorption of dietary fat.
- Contributes to weight loss and improvements in metabolic parameters such as:
  - HbA1c
  - LDL cholesterol
  - Total cholesterol
- Meta-analysis showed a mean weight loss of 8% compared to placebo groups and sustained weight loss with continuous therapy for up to 36 months.
- Beneficial for patients with coronary artery disease or other cardiac conditions since Orlistat offers a weight loss option with a relatively favorable cardiovascular safety profile.
- Common adverse effects include:
  - Uncontrollable stools
  - Flatulence
  - Oily stools
- Potential deficiencies in fat-soluble vitamins and minerals, requiring supplementary vitamin intake. Naltrexone/Bupropion Extended-Release (Contrave)
- FDA-approved in 2014.
- Initial dosing starts at 8/90 mg daily.
- The dose progressively increases over 4 weeks.
- Bupropion works as a dopamine and norepinephrine reuptake inhibitor and is used primarily for smoking cessation and depression.
- Naltrexone works as an opioid receptor antagonist and is used in the treatment of opioid and alcohol dependence.
- The combination is hypothesized to act on the hypothalamus to:
  - Enhance satiety
  - Decrease food intake
  - Elevate energy expenditure
- Clinical trials have demonstrated a weight reduction of around 5%.
- Potential for up to a 9.2% decrease when used in conjunction with intensive behavioral therapy.
- Side effects include:
  - Nausea
  - Constipation
  - Headache
  - Anxiety

- Suitable for patients with comorbid depression.
- Should be avoided in individuals with due bupropion lowering the seizure threshold:
  - Uncontrolled hypertension
  - Bulimia nervosa
  - Seizures
  - History of alcohol withdrawal

Gelesis100
- First anti-obesity agent approved by the FDA for adults with overweight (BMI 25–40 kg/m^2), regardless of comorbidities.
- Classified as a medical device rather than a drug due to its mechanical mode of action.
- Consists of a hydrogel matrix made from modified cellulose cross-linked with citric acid.
- Upon ingestion, it absorbs water and expands to occupy approximately one-fourth of the average stomach volume.
- Promotes a sensation of fullness, helping to reduce overall food intake.
- The recommended dosage is 6.75 mg which is taken with 500 ml of water 20–30 min before meals.
- Operates purely through physical means rather than systemic effects [1–6].

Site of action of FDA approved anti-obesity medications

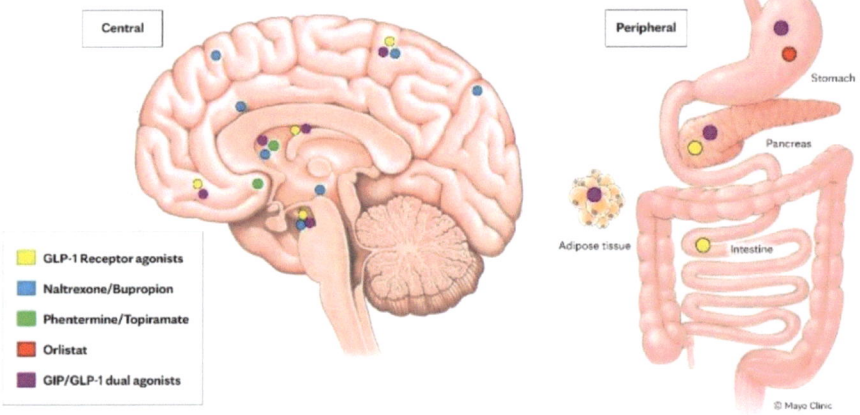

Endoscopic Sleeve Gastroplasty (ESG)

Lindsey Trinchet and Fernando Elli

Introduction

Endoscopic sleeve gastroplasty (ESG), also known as the "Apollo method," is a weight-loss procedure that shortens and reshapes the gastric body into a "sleeve". The tubular shape delays gastric emptying and restricts volume intake. The anterior and posterior walls are bound together along the greater curvature by 6–12 running stitches using full-thickness endoscopic suturing device [7–10].

Indications

- Patients with a BMI above 27 kg/m^2; a BMI of 30–40 kg/m^2, is ideal for ESG.
- ESG is appropriate for obese patients who do not qualify for bariatric surgery [7–10].

Contraindications

- Gastric ulcers and congestive gastropathy are considered absolute contraindications.
- Patients with gastric polyposis and gastric or esophageal varices have an greater risk of bleeding.
- Hiatal hernias increase risk of injury to surrounding organs and structures in the thorax (Fig. 7.1) [7–10].

Outcomes

- Estimated weight loss is 18–20% at 1 year when combined with lifestyle modifications; 12–20% at 5 years.
- At 5 years, most patients maintain ≥10% weight loss.
- Most patients report remission or improvement of hypertension, type 2 diabetes, and dyslipidemia.
- ESG has not been shown to impact nutrient or hormone levels [7–10].

Fig. 7.1 Stomach before and after ESG

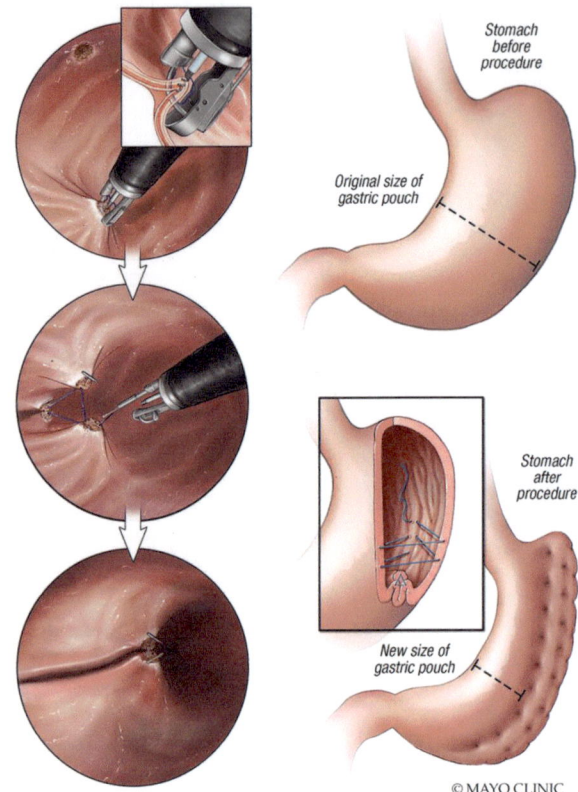

How the stitches are placed (left images); before and after images of the stomach.

Complications

- Mild adverse symptoms (nausea vomiting, pain) are common.
- Severe complications (bleeding/perforation, abscess, damage to surrounding organs) are rare (0.8–2.8%) [7–10].

Intragastric Balloons

Isabella Reitz and Fernando Elli

Introduction

In patients with obesity who have not succeeded with conventional weight-loss methods, intragastric balloon therapy can be combined with lifestyle modifications as a weight-loss strategy. Intragastric balloon therapy is a minimally invasive and temporary method that involves placing a saline- or air-filled balloon in the stomach, typically through endoscopy. Three FDA-approved intragastric balloons include Orbera, Reshape, and Obalon [11–13].

History of Intra-Gastric Balloons

- The first intragastric balloon, the Garren-Edwards Gastric Bubble (GEGB), was introduced in 1985 by gastroenterologists Lloyd and Mary Garren.
- The GEGB was a cylindrical balloon filled with 200 mL of air and was designed to remain in the stomach for 4 months.
- Although it received FDA approval, the GEGB was withdrawn in 1992 due to complications such as gastric ulcers, Mallory-Weiss tears, small bowel obstructions, and inadequate weight loss results.
- In 1987, an international consensus established specifications for balloon safety and design, including:
  - Smooth surfaces
  - Durable materials
  - Liquid filling
  - Radiopaque markers
  - Adjustable sizes
- In 1991, BioEnterics Corporation developed a saline-filled balloon known as Orbera.
- The Orbera balloon received FDA approval in 2015.
- Since then, various intragastric balloon systems have been introduced to the market [11–13].

How Intragastric Balloons Function

- Weight Loss is achieved through restriction and the sensation of satiation by occupying up to one-third of the stomach cavity, which limits caloric intake.
- Balloon placement significantly slows the gastric emptying of solids and liquids after 3 months.

- Individuals with high liquid calorie intake may experience less benefit from intragastric balloon therapy.
- Afferent cells from the gastrointestinal tract and adipose tissue send signals to the brainstem, which processes hunger, satiety, and satiation. Stomach distention activates this system.
- Studies show that balloon-induced distention affects brain regions involved in pain processing. This pain processing is part of visceral pain and is reduced with nutrient infusion, potentially to ensure adequate nutritional intake despite extensive stomach extension [11–13].

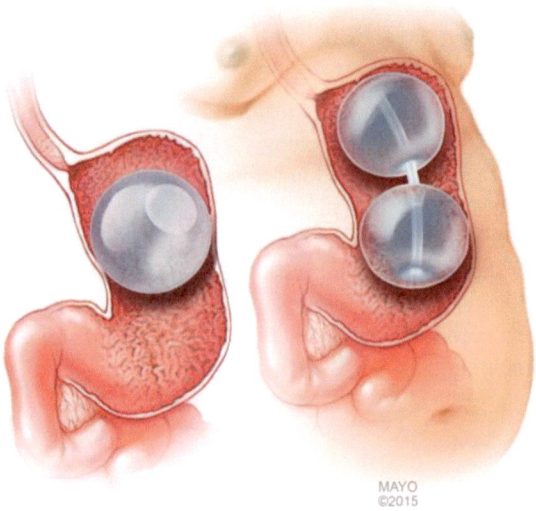

Indications

- Intragastric balloon therapy is indicated for individuals with a Body Mass Index (BMI) of 30–35 kg/m^2 who have not achieved sufficient weight loss through other methods.

Contraindications

- Relative contraindications for intra-gastric balloon therapy include:
- Large hiatal hernia (≥3 cm)
- Inflammatory bowel diseases (e.g., ulcerative colitis, Crohn's disease)

- Previous abdominal surgeries
- Esophagitis
- Chronic use of nonsteroidal anti-inflammatory drugs (NSAIDs)
- Uncontrolled psychiatric disorders
- Psychiatric disorders should be managed before balloon placement to ensure patient compliance and successful therapy outcomes.
- Absolute contraindications for intra-gastric balloon therapy include:
- Hiatal hernia larger than 5 cm (specifically for the Orbera balloon) [11–13]

Procedure

- Intragastric balloon placement is an outpatient procedure typically conducted in an endoscopy unit, lasting about 30 min, with the patient generally being discharged 1 to 2 h afterward.
- The procedure begins with light sedation, usually with propofol, followed by an endoscopic evaluation of the lower esophagus and stomach to detect ulcers or large hiatal hernias.
- The deflated balloon is then inserted into the stomach through the esophagus under endoscopic guidance. Once correctly positioned, the balloon is inflated with fluid in 50 mL increments, up to a maximum of 500 mL, and has a self-sealing valve to prevent leaks.
- Balloon removal is performed in the endoscopy suite under light sedation, where the balloon is punctured with a needle, deflated, and then extracted through the mouth using a grasper [11–13].

Complications

- Early complications of intragastric balloon therapy include:
- 7.2% of patients requiring treatment for dehydration
- 2% of patients needing readmission
- 1.1% of patients requiring re-operation
- Gastrointestinal symptoms are common and may affect up to 91% of patients, including nausea, abdominal pain, vomiting, dyspepsia, constipation, acid reflux, and burping.
- To manage these symptoms, proton pump inhibitors, anti-emetics (e.g., ondansetron, aprepitant), and anticholinergics (e.g., scopolamine) are used, especially in the first week.
- About 4–7% of patients experience significant symptoms beyond the first week, with less than 3% potentially needing endoscopic re-intervention or early balloon removal.

- Serious events associated with intragastric balloons include gastric perforation (~0.1%), balloon rupture and migration (~1.4%), acute pancreatitis (more common with liquid-filled balloons), and spontaneous hyperinflation, which is mainly reported with the Orbera balloon and may necessitate early removal.
- Mortality rates are reported between 0.05 and 0.08%, with causes including esophageal perforation, pulmonary embolism, gastric perforation, and unknown factors [11–13].

Outcomes

- Initial weight loss from intragastric balloon therapy typically results in a 6–15% total body weight reduction, compared to 1–5% through lifestyle changes alone.
- Long-term results show that only 50% of patients maintain 20% excess weight loss at 1-year post-removal. Only 25% of patients maintain 20% excess weight loss at 5 years.

References

1. Abdi Beshir S, Ahmed Elnour A, Soorya A, Parveen Mohamed A, Sir Loon Goh S, Hussain N, Al Haddad AHI, Hussain F, Yousif Khidir I, Abdelnassir Z. A narrative review of approved and emerging anti-obesity medications. Saudi Pharm J. 2023;31(10):101757. https://doi.org/10.1016/j.jsps.2023.101757.
2. Tchang BG, Aras M, Kumar RB, et al. Pharmacologic treatment of overweight and obesity in adults. 2024. MDText.com. Available from: https://www.ncbi.nlm.nih.gov/books/NBK279038/
3. Tak YJ, Lee SY. Long-term efficacy and safety of anti-obesity treatment: where do we stand? Curr Obes Rep. 2021;10(1):14–30.
4. Rodrigues Silva Sombra L, Anastasopoulou C. Pharmacologic therapy for obesity. Treasure Island: StatPearls; 2024.
5. Perreault L, Reid TJ. Obesity in adults: drug therapy. Waltham: UpToDate; 2024.
6. Jensterle M, Rizzo M, Haluzík M, Janež A. Efficacy of GLP-1 RA approved for weight management in patients with or without diabetes: a narrative review. Adv Ther. 2022;39(6):2452–67.
7. Brunaldi VO, Neto MG. Endoscopic sleeve gastroplasty: a narrative review on historical evolution, physiology, outcomes, and future standpoints. Chin Med J. 2022;135(7):774–8.
8. Docimo S Jr, Aylward L, Albaugh VL, Afaneh C, El Djouzi S, Ali M, Altieri MS, Carter J. American Society for Metabolic and Bariatric Surgery Clinical Issues Committee. Endoscopic sleeve gastroplasty and its role in the treatment of obesity: a systematic review. Surg Obes Relat Dis. 2023;19(11):1205–18.
9. Mayo Clinic. Endoscopic sleeve gastroplasty. 2019. Available from: https://www.mayoclinic.org/tests-procedures/endoscopic-sleeve-gastroplasty/about/pac-20393958.

10. Corl FM. Stomach before and after endoscopic sleeve gastroplasty. Mayo Clinic Media Archives. 2015. MC1996-08. Available from: https://mcmedia.mayo.edu/asset-management/241HRGTJ7FXM?WS=SearchResults
11. Crossan K, Sheer AJ. Intragastric balloon. In: StatPearls [Internet]. Treasure Island: StatPearls; 2023. Publishing; Available from: https://www.ncbi.nlm.nih.gov/books/NBK578184/.
12. Stavrou G, Shrewsbury A, Kotzampassi K. Six intragastric balloons: which to choose? World J Gastrointest Endosc. 2021;13(8):238–59.
13. Muniraj T, Day LW, Teigen LM, Ho EY, Sultan S, Davitkov P, Shah R, Murad MH. AGA clinical practice guidelines on intragastric balloons in the management of obesity. Gastroenterology. 2021;160(5):1799–808.

Index

A
Adjustable gastric band (AGB), 8, 35–40, 42–52
Alternatives, 77–88
Anesthesia, 25, 27–33, 36

B
Bariatric surgery, 5–12, 21–33, 35, 40, 55–73, 77–88
  candidate, 21–23
Biliary disease, 60
Biliopancreatic diversion (BPD), 9–11, 23, 40, 46–52, 57, 63
Bypass, 6–9, 11, 23, 43, 45–48, 52, 56–59, 66, 70

C
Comorbidities, 22–25, 27, 28, 31, 43, 45, 52, 77, 82
Coronary heart disease (CHD), 15, 16, 18, 80
Counseling, 21, 23–27

D
Diabetes, 2, 11, 20, 22, 24, 26–28, 39, 43, 45, 52, 67, 69, 78, 83
Dumping syndrome, 11, 45, 47, 64–66

E
Education, 23–27
Endoscopic sleeve gastroplasty (ESG), 83–84

Epidemic, 2
Evolution, 12

F
Fistulas, 68–73

G
Gastric sleeve, 9, 42, 48, 50, 57

H
History, 5–12, 28, 60, 67, 69, 82, 85
Hyperlipidemia, 15, 18, 24, 52
Hypertension, 16–18, 24, 26–28, 36, 43, 45, 52, 69, 80, 82, 83

I
Incidence, 1–2, 7, 11, 42, 47, 52, 62, 64, 68, 71, 72
Internal hernia, 45, 50, 52, 71
Intragastric balloons, 85–86, 88

L
Leaks, 10, 39, 68–73, 87

M
Marginal ulcers, 66–68
Multi-disciplinary, 23

N
Nutrition, 2, 5, 12, 26, 63, 69

O
Obesity, 1, 2, 5, 11, 12, 15–24, 27, 28, 30, 33, 60, 77, 78, 85

P
Physiology, 15–20, 61
Prevalence, 1–2, 66

S
Steatotic liver disease, 19
Surgical technique, 36–38, 40–46, 49–51

V
Venous thromboembolism (VTE), 31, 72, 73

W
Weight loss medications, 77

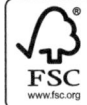

If you have any concerns about our products,
you can contact us on
ProductSafety@springernature.com

In case Publisher is established outside the EU,
the EU authorized representative is:
Springer Nature Customer Service Center GmbH
Europaplatz 3, 69115 Heidelberg, Germany

Printed by Libri Plureos GmbH
in Hamburg, Germany